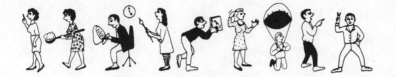

The Enneagram Made Easy

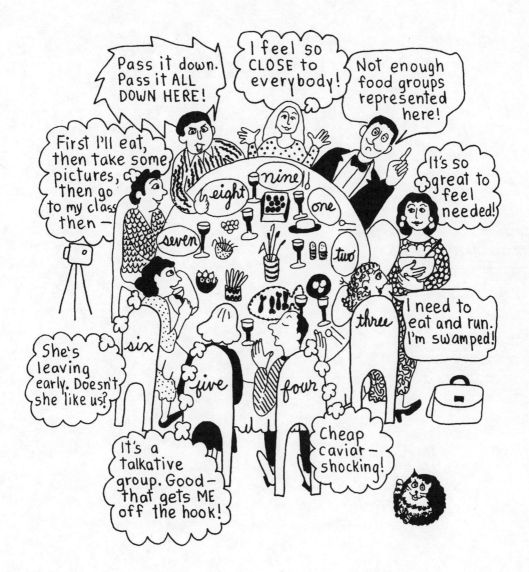

The Enneagram Made Easy

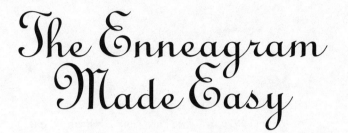

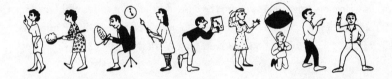

Discover the 9 Types of People

Renee Baron &
Elizabeth Wagele

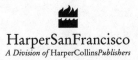

HarperSanFrancisco
A Division of HarperCollinsPublishers

FIRST EDITION

Library of Congress Cataloging-in-Publication Data:

Baron, Renee.
The enneagram made easy : discover the nine types of people /
Renee Baron & Elizabeth Wagele. — 1st ed.
     p.   cm.
Includes bibliographic references.
ISBN 0–06–251026–6 (alk. paper)
     1. Enneagram.   I. Wagele, Elizabeth.   II. Title.
BF698.35.E54B37 1994   93–31824
155.2'6—dc20   CIP

94 95 96 97 98 ❖ RRD(H) 10 9 8 7 6 5 4 3

This edition is printed on acid-free paper that meets the
American National Standards Institute Z39.48 Standard.

To Liz (a Five) for all the years of laughter and
friendship, and for your ability to get to the kernel of truth in
your writing. To my children: Jodi, Tami, and Dan, and to my friends, with
thanks for your love and support. With gratitude to the Twelve-Step
community and the guidance of my Higher Power.
—Renee

To Renee (a Two) for your friendship,
wit, and knowledge, and most of all for your honesty.
Also to my family: Gus, Nick, Martha, Augie, and
Miranda, and friends. Thanks for your help.
—Liz

This book was illustrated by Liz with
Renee looking over her shoulder and is proof that
any two people can work together using the Enneagram.

Contents

Enneagram

The Enneagram is a study of the nine basic types of people. It explains why we behave the way we do, and it points to specific directions for individual growth. It is an important tool for improving relationships with family, friends, and co-workers.

The roots of the Enneagram go back many centuries. Its exact origin is not known, but it is believed to have been taught orally in secret Sufi brotherhoods in the Middle East. The Russian mystical teacher G. I. Gurdjieff introduced it to Europe in the 1920s, and it arrived in the United States in the 1960s.

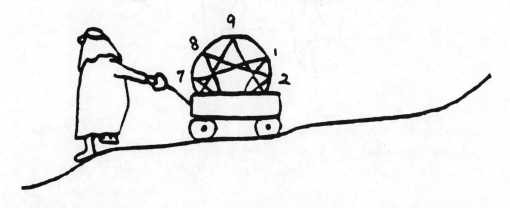

The Enneagram (pronounced ANY-a-gram) system is represented by a circle containing a nine-pointed starlike shape. *Ennea* is Greek for the number nine, and *gram* means "a drawing." *Enneagram* means "a drawing with nine points."

The Enneagram teaches that early in life we learned to feel safe and to cope with our family situations and personal circumstances by developing a strategy based on our natural talents and abilities.

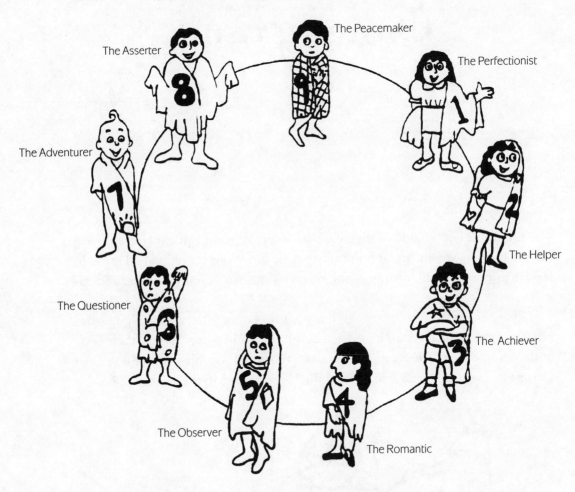

By working with the Enneagram we develop a deeper understanding of others and learn alternatives to our own patterns of behavior. We break free from worn-out coping strategies and begin to see life from a broader point of view.

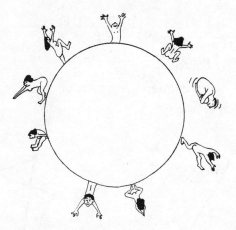

People of the same type have the same basic motivations and view the world in some fundamentally similar ways. Variations within each type stem from such factors as maturity, parents' types, birth order, cultural values, and inherent traits such as being naturally introverted or extroverted.

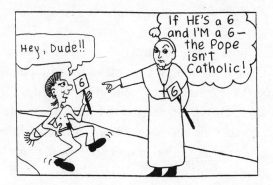

As you learn the Enneagram, you will readily begin to "type" people you know. We urge you to keep your guesses to yourself and to keep an open mind. Deciding one's type accurately is important and must be done by each person according to his or her own internal perception.

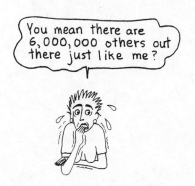

It may be a comfort to know that millions of people have the same coping strategy as you. The behavior patterns that emerge from the nine types are, however, as numerous, mysterious, and unique as the individuals involved.

Moving Around the Enneagram

1. The Enneagram Drawing

The nine points on the circumference of the circle are divided into a triangle and a six-pointed shape:

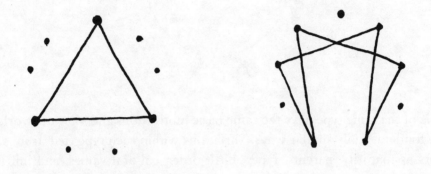

2. The Arrows

Each point on the Enneagram connects to two other points. These two points or types are called your arrows. When relaxed, you take on the positive qualities of the number that connects to yours in this order: 1–7–5–8–2–4–1 and 3–6–9–3. One goes to Seven, Seven goes to Five, and so on. When under stress, you reverse directions: One takes on the negative qualities of Four, Four of Two, and so on. The arrows are a dynamic tool for personal growth and are explained in each chapter.

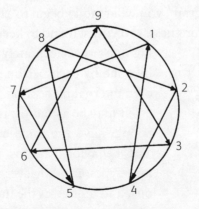

3. The Wings

Your personality may blend into or be influenced by the types on either side of yours. For instance, a Nine may have some characteristics of a One or an Eight. These neighboring types are called your wings.

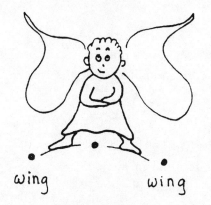

wing   wing

Some people seem to have been different types as children than as adults. Usually these types are related by the arrows or wings.

A Brief Description of the Nine Types

1. *Perfectionists* are realistic, conscientious, and principled. They strive to live up to their high ideals.

2. *Helpers* are warm, concerned, nurturing, and sensitive to other people's needs.

3. *Achievers* are energetic, optimistic, self-assured, and goal oriented.

4. *Romantics* have sensitive feelings and are warm and perceptive.

5. *Observers* have a need for knowledge and are introverted, curious, analytical, and insightful.

6. *Questioners* are responsible, trustworthy, and value loyalty to family, friends, groups, and causes. Their personalities range broadly from reserved and timid to outspoken and confrontative.

7. *Adventurers* are energetic, lively, and optimistic. They want to contribute to the world.

8. *Asserters* are direct, self-reliant, self-confident, and protective.

9. *Peacemakers* are receptive, good-natured, and supportive. They seek union with others and the world around them.

The Three Centers

Finding your "center" is a key to finding your type. Each center is made up of three adjacent types, corresponding to the three centers of the body: the heart, the head, and the gut.

The Heart or Feeling Center (Image)

Helpers (Twos) are interested in people and in nurturing. They want to present a loving image.

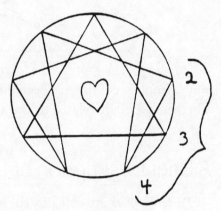

Achievers (Threes) like to be seen in a good light, according to socially agreed-upon norms.

Romantics (Fours) have strong needs to express themselves and to be seen as original.

The Head or Thinking Center (Fear)

Observers (Fives) rely on their own resources and find safety in knowledge.

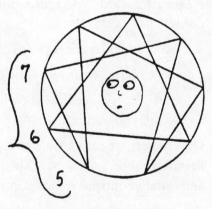

Questioners (Sixes) seek relief from fear through the permission and approval of authority figures or through rebelling against authority.

Adventurers (Sevens) are active and optimistic. They shun unpleasant emotions, including fear.

The Gut or Instinctive Center (Anger)

Asserters (Eights) present a strong image and are not afraid to express their anger.

Peacemakers (Nines) are agreeable, accommodating, and can often be out of touch with their anger.

Perfectionists (Ones) see anger as a character flaw and try to hold it back. They follow standards of behavior closely and/or try to better the world.

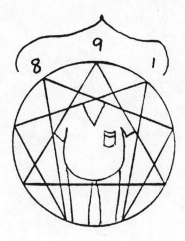

How to Find Your Type

Along with looking for your center, here are other ways to search for your type.

1. The Personality Inventories

Fill out the inventories at the beginning of each chapter. Answer the questions according to what you were like when you were (or if you are now) under the age of 25, when behavior habits are the most automatic. The inventory you score highest on *may* be your type, but don't stop there. It is best to read all the chapters and take all the inventories. If you can't decide between two adjacent numbers, one may be your more developed wing.

2. The Comparison of the Enneagram with the Jungian Types

The final chapter briefly explains the Myers-Briggs inventory of Jungian types and compares the two systems. It expands the dimensions of the Enneagram and can also help you find your type.

Remember, you are the only one who can decide on your type. Don't accept being "typed" by others.

BEFORE THE DINNER PARTY

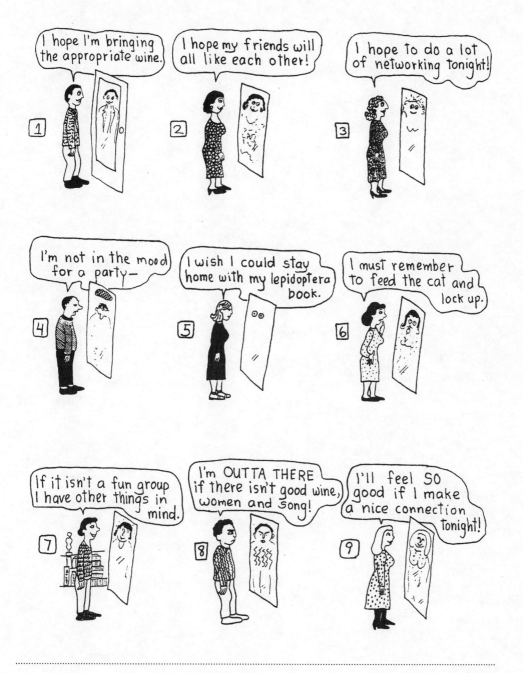

THE

Perfectionist

I may have faults, but being wrong ain't one of them.
—Jimmy Hoffa

Ones are motivated by the need to live their life the right way, including improving themselves and the world around them.

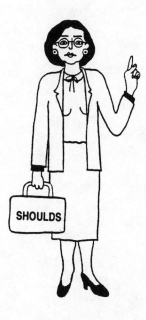

Ones at their BEST are	Ones at their WORST are
ethical	judgmental
reliable	inflexible
productive	dogmatic
wise	obsessive-compulsive
idealistic	critical of others
fair	overly serious
honest	controlling
orderly	anxious
self-disciplined	jealous

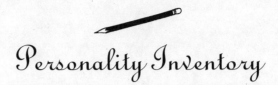

Personality Inventory

Check what describes you when you were (or if you are now) under the age of 25.

- [ ] 1   I like to be organized and orderly.
- [ ] 2   It is difficult for me to be spontaneous.
- [ ] 3   I often feel guilty about not getting enough accomplished.
- [ ] 4   I don't like it when people break rules.
- [x] 5   Incorrect grammar and spelling bother me a lot.
- [x] 6   I am idealistic. I want to make the world a better place.
- [x] 7   I am almost always on time.
- [ ] 8   I hold on to resentment for a long time.
- [x] 9   I think of myself as being practical, reasonable, and realistic.
- [ ] 10   When jealous, I become fearful and competitive.
- [ ] 11   Either I don't have enough time to relax or I think I shouldn't relax.
- [ ] 12   I tend to see things in terms of right or wrong, good or bad.
- [ ] 13   I analyze major purchases very thoroughly before I make them.
- [ ] 14   I dread being criticized or judged by others.
- [ ] 15   I often compare myself with others.
- [ ] 16   Truth and justice are very important to me.
- [ ] 17   I often feel that time is running out and there is too much left to do.
- [ ] 18   I almost always do what I say I will do.
- [ ] 19   I worry almost constantly.
- [ ] 20   I love making every detail perfect.

4

Perfectionist (1)

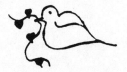

How to Get Along with Me

- Take your share of the responsibility so I don't end up with all the work.
- Acknowledge my achievements.
- I'm hard on myself. Reassure me that I'm fine the way I am.
- Tell me that you value my advice.
- Be fair and considerate, as I am.
- Apologize if you have been unthoughtful. It will help me to forgive.
- Gently encourage me to lighten up and to laugh at myself when I get uptight, but hear my worries first.

Relationships

Ones at their best in a relationship are loyal, dedicated, conscientious, and helpful. They are well balanced and have a good sense of humor.

 Ones at their worst in a relationship are critical, argumentative, nit-picking, and uncompromising. They have high expectations of others.

What I Like About Being a One

- being self-disciplined and able to accomplish a great deal
- working hard to make the world a better place
- having high standards and ethics; not compromising myself
- being reasonable, responsible, and dedicated in everything I do
- being able to put facts together, coming to good understandings, and figuring out wise solutions
- being the best I can be and bringing out the best in other people

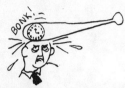

What's Hard About Being a One

- being disappointed with myself or others when my expectations are not met
- feeling burdened by too much responsibility
- thinking that what I do is never good enough
- not being appreciated for what I do for people
- being upset because others aren't trying as hard as I am
- obsessing about what I did or what I should do
- being tense, anxious, and taking things too seriously

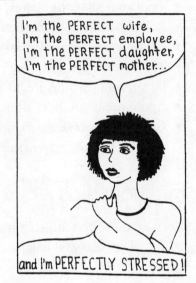

How I Drive Myself Crazy

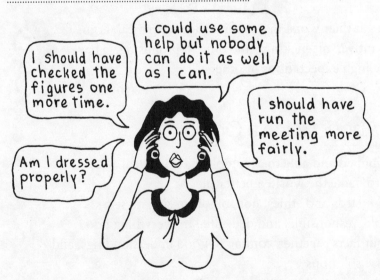

Ones as Children Often

- criticize themselves in anticipation of criticism from others
- refrain from doing things that they think might not come out perfect
- focus on living up to the expectations of their parents and teachers
- are very responsible; may assume the role of parent
- hold back negative emotions ("good children aren't angry")

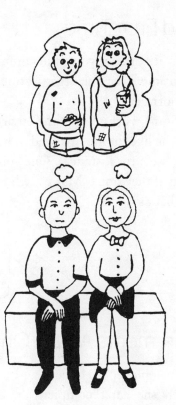

Ones as Parents

- teach their children responsibility and strong moral values
- are consistent and fair
- discipline firmly

Careers

Ones are efficient, organized, and always complete the task. The more analytical and tough-minded Ones are found in management, science, and law enforcement. The more people-oriented Ones are found in health care, education, and religious work.

Since they do things in a professional, honest, and ethical manner, you would do well to have Ones as your car mechanic, surgeon, dentist, banker, and stockbroker.

And Free Time

Ones are often involved in community service groups (PTAs, scouts, neighborhood improvement organizations, etc.). Many have *Robert's Rules of Order* memorized.

Some work to save the environment through the Sierra Club, Greenpeace, and the like, or are involved in humanitarian causes (on either side of the abortion issue, for instance). Ones often work out and diet for good health, or feel guilty if they don't. Many are busy helping friends and family. Ones are usually excellent students.

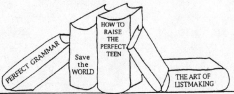

Comments About Ones

"My employee is efficient and patient. When she can't complete an assignment, she'll take it home. If she ever leaves, I'll have to hire two people to take her place."

"My friend quit his job because his boss wanted him to do something that was unethical. He is committed to living by his principles and will never sacrifice his morals. He practices what he preaches."

"My One friend is a teacher. It's hard on her because she is determined to read every single word of every paper and write down every criticism possible. The students love her because she is interesting, inspiring, and fair."

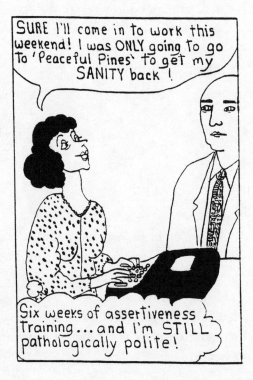

"When I need help with anything, he's always ready to lend me a hand. He stays until the job is completely finished."

Wings

Your personality may blend into or be influenced by the types on either side of yours. A strong wing can make a big difference in your personality.

Ones with a more developed Two wing tend to be warmer, more helpful, critical, and controlling.

Ones with a more developed Nine wing tend to be cooler, more relaxed, objective, and detached.

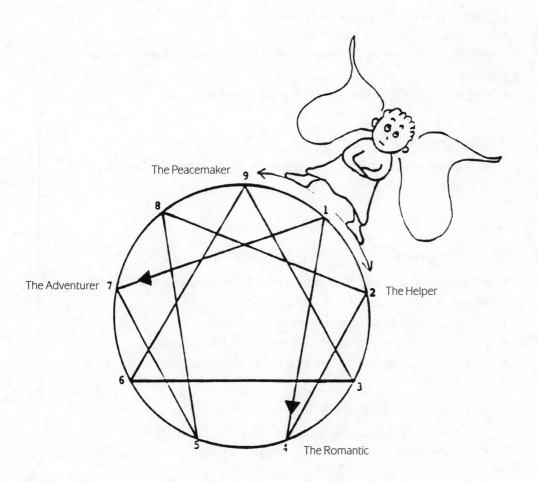

Moving Around Within the Enneagram

Following the lines in the diagram, the One moves toward Seven in one direction and toward Four in the other. Ones move toward the positive side of Seven when they feel secure; they can also consciously cultivate these positive qualities. Ones move toward the negative side of Four when in stress; they can consciously try to avoid these negative traits. Read the chapters about types Four and Seven to learn more about them.

When Ones Move Toward the Positive Side of Seven They

- become less self-critical and more self-accepting
- become more enthusiastic and optimistic
- act more naturally and spontaneously
- shift their attitude away from what's bad in the situation toward what's good
- plan more activities that are simply for enjoyment

When Ones Move to the Negative Side of Seven They

- become self-destructive through substance abuse or other excessive behavior

When Ones Move Toward the Negative Side of Four They

- feel indignant because their expectations are not being met by themselves, others, or life in general
- turn their anger inward and become depressed
- lose trust in themselves and/or feel unloved and unlovable
- long for what they don't have and feel hopeless about ever getting it

When Ones Move to the Positive Side of Four They

- get in touch with deeper feelings
- become involved in creative or artistic activities

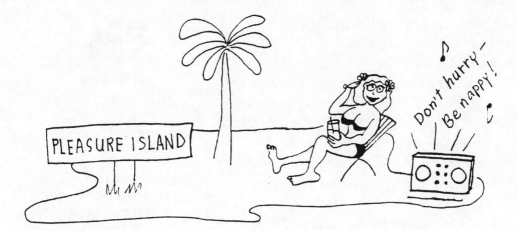

Practical Suggestions and Exercises for a One

1. Self-Nurturing

- Spend some time each day doing some recreational activities you enjoy, for instance, gardening, watching movies, playing a sport, walking, being with friends, or puttering in your workshop.
- Give yourself special treats regularly (flowers, sports events, bubble baths, dinner at your favorite restaurant).
- Accentuate the importance of humor in your life. Memorize jokes, collect cartoons, watch comedy shows.
- Become aware of what you want and learn to ask for it (even for whims).
- Avoid the word *should*. Change the should sentence to "I *want* to . . . " or "I *don't want* to. . . ." For example, "I should visit Mike" becomes "I want to visit Mike" or "I don't want to visit Mike."
- Take a class in and practice stress reduction, meditation, or yoga.
- Pat yourself on the back for allowing yourself to have one helter-skelter drawer, closet, or room.
- Take vacations to get away from work and compulsive doing.

2. Recognizing and Working with Anger

- Be aware that you may make sarcastic or cynical remarks when you feel hurt and defensive.

- Learn to accept anger as a normal and useful human emotion.
- Ask yourself if there is something you haven't been aware of beneath your anger, such as sadness or disappointment.
- Try to realize that expressing anger will not make you unlovable.
- If expressing your feelings directly does not seem appropriate, exercise, write, or talk with a friend.
- You will become more frustrated and angrier if you pressure yourself and others to live up to unrealistic expectations.

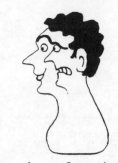

Sometimes Ones have a smile on their face, but they're seething underneath.

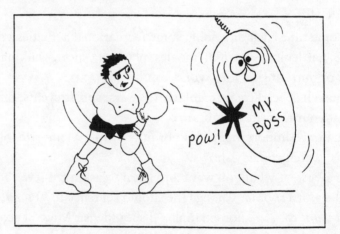

Find a safe outlet for your anger.

3. Work

- Evaluate your job and make sure it is appropriate for you and fulfilling.
- Ask others to help so you don't do more than your share. If you are afraid they won't do it as well as you, find another One to do the job!
- Allow yourself to do certain things quickly, although imperfectly, so you can get on to the next task or go home on time.
- Instead of mentally rehashing past mistakes, remember the accomplishments you are most proud of.

- Don't let one flaw in your performance make you feel worthless.
- Be willing to drop down a few notches from being perfect.

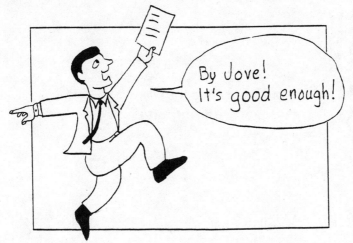

4. Relationships

There is so much good in the worst of us and so much bad in the best of us, that it's rather hard to tell which of us ought to reform the rest of us.

—Sign in Springdale, Connecticut

- Learn to forgive yourself and others for flaws and mistakes.
- Learn to respect others' ways of doing things that are different from yours.
- Be generous with praise and encouragement.
- When you get the urge to criticize or correct someone, either keep quiet or surround what you say with positive (not flattering!) remarks.
- Become aware that your tone of voice can be harsh and can upset or frighten people.
- Avoid fantasizing about changing people.

For Parents

- Allow your children to come to decisions on their own in order for them to develop more self-esteem.
- Let your children know you love them not only for what they do, but for who they are.

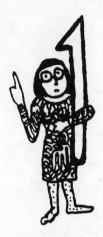

See everything;
overlook a great deal;
correct a little.

—Pope John XXIII

I have found the best way to give advice
to your children is to find out what they want
and then advise them to do it.

—Harry Truman

Things Ones Would Never Dream of Doing

- being half an hour late to work
- not sending thank-you notes for birthday gifts within two days
- not making reservations for every night of their vacation
- leaving their clothes in a heap and their dishes unwashed all week
- laughing it off when criticized
- eating with their elbows on the table and using their sleeve for a napkin
- taking a relaxing bath just before guests come over instead of going over the house for another cleaning

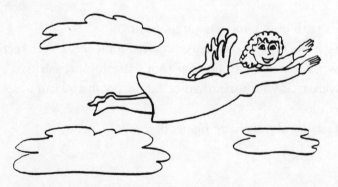

Angels fly because they take themselves lightly.

Positive Things to Say to Yourself

It is OK to relax and enjoy myself.

I'm OK even when I make mistakes.

I am learning not to take myself so seriously.

I am perfect just the way I am.

I will ask for what I want and need.

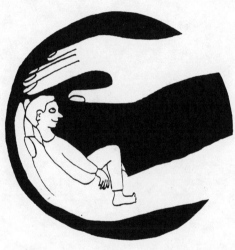

Thou Shalt Not Should on Thyself

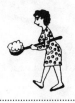

THE

Helper

We are all here on earth to help others;
what on earth the others are here for I don't know.
—W. H. Auden

Twos are motivated by the need to be loved and valued and to express their positive feelings toward others.

Traditionally society has encouraged Two qualities in females more than in males.

Twos at their BEST are	Twos at their WORST are
loving	martyrlike
caring	indirect
adaptable	manipulative
insightful	possessive
generous	hysterical
enthusiastic	overly accommodating
tuned in to how people feel	overly demonstrative (the more extroverted Twos)

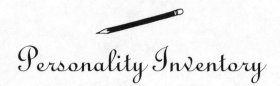

Personality Inventory

Check what describes you when you were (or if you are now) under the age of 25.

- ☐ 1 I want people to feel comfortable coming to me for guidance and advice.
- ☐ 2 Relationships are more important to me than almost anything.
- ☐ 3 Sometimes I feel overburdened by people's dependence on me.
- ☐ 4 I have trouble asking for what I need.
- ☐ 5 I crave, yet sometimes fear, intimacy.
- ☐ 6 I am more comfortable giving than receiving.
- ☐ 7 I am very sensitive to criticism.
- ☐ 8 I work hard to overcome all obstacles in a relationship.
- ☐ 9 I try to be as sensitive and tactful as possible.
- ☐ 10 When I am alone I know what I want, but when I am with others I am not sure.
- ☐ 11 It is very important that others feel comfortable and welcome in my home.
- ☐ 12 I don't want my dependence to show.
- ☐ 13 Watching violence on television and seeing people suffer is unbearable.
- ☐ 14 Sometimes I feel a deep sense of loneliness.
- ☐ 15 If I don't get the closeness I need, I feel sad, hurt, and unimportant.
- ☐ 16 Sometimes I get physically ill and emotionally drained from taking care of everyone else.
- ☐ 17 I often figure out what others would like in a person, then act that way.
- ☐ 18 I enjoy giving compliments and telling people that they are special to me.
- ☐ 19 I am attracted to being with important or powerful people.
- ☐ 20 People have said I exaggerate too much and am overly emotional.

7

Helper (2)

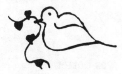

How to Get Along with Me

- Tell me that you appreciate me. Be specific.
- Share fun times with me.
- Take an interest in my problems, though I will probably try to focus on yours.
- Let me know that I am important and special to you.
- Be gentle if you decide to criticize me.

In Intimate Relationships

- Reassure me that I am interesting to you.
- Reassure me often that you love me.
- Tell me I'm attractive and that you're glad to be seen with me.

Relationships

Twos at their best in a relationship are attentive, appreciative, generous, warm, playful, and nurturing. Twos make their partners feel special and loved.

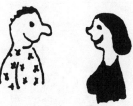

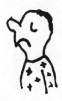

Twos at their worst in a relationship are controlling, possessive, needy, and insincere. Since they have trouble asking directly, they tend to manipulate to get what they want.

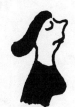

What I Like About Being a Two

- being able to relate easily to people and to make friends
- knowing what people need and being able to make their lives better
- being generous, caring, and warm
- being sensitive to and perceptive about others' feelings
- being enthusiastic and fun-loving, and having a good sense of humor

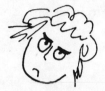

What's Hard About Being a Two

- not being able to say no
- having low self-esteem
- feeling drained from overdoing for others
- not doing things I really like to do for myself for fear of being selfish
- criticizing myself for not feeling as loving as I think I should
- being upset that others don't tune in to me as much as I tune in to them
- working so hard to be tactful and considerate that I suppress my real feelings

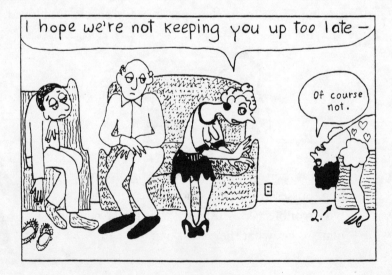

Typical Thoughts of a Two

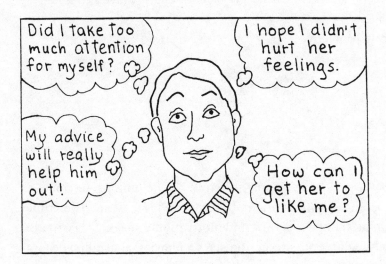

Twos as Children Often

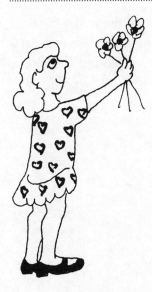

- are very sensitive to disapproval and criticism
- try hard to please their parents by being helpful and understanding
- are outwardly compliant
- are popular or try to be popular with other children
- act coy, precocious, or dramatic in order to get attention
- are clowns and jokers (the more extroverted Twos), or quiet and shy (the more introverted Twos)

Twos as Parents

- are good listeners, love their children unconditionally, and are warm and encouraging (or suffer guilt if they aren't)

- are often playful with their children
- wonder: "Am I doing it right?" "Am I giving enough?" "Have I caused irreparable damage?"
- can become fiercely protective

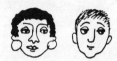

Careers

Twos usually prefer to work with people, often in the helping professions, as counselors, teachers, and health workers. Extroverted Twos are sometimes found in the limelight as actresses, actors, and motivational speakers. Twos also work in sales and helping others as receptionists, secretaries, assistants, decorators, and clothing consultants.

And Free Time

Twos enjoy socializing with family or friends, caring for children, making their homes warm and inviting, gardening, reading, working for charitable organizations, having new experiences in the outside world, and exploring their inner world.

Many Twos take special care of their appearance.

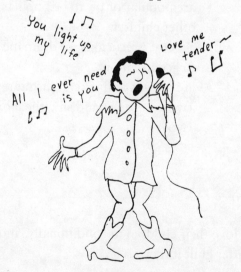

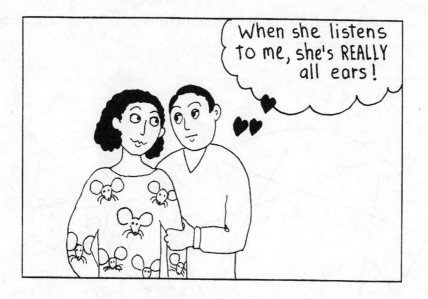

Comments About Twos

"She is loved by many because she gives so generously of herself. When a friend had cancer, she was the main support system for the family while still managing to put energy into her career."

"My Two friends are easy for me to be around. They are lighthearted and playful as well as having tremendous depth and wisdom. I wish I could articulate my feelings as well as they can."

"He is a wonderful father. He showers his children with attention, generosity, and love."

"When I have a problem, I call my Two friend. She's always perceptive, sympathetic, and nonjudgmental."

Wings

Your personality may blend into or be influenced by the types on either side of yours. A strong wing can make a big difference in your personality.

Twos with a stronger One wing tend to be more idealistic, objective, self-critical, and judgmental.

Twos with a stronger Three wing tend to be more self-assured, ambitious, outgoing, and competitive.

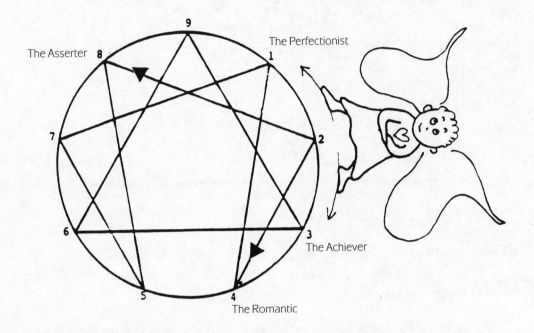

The Perfectionist

The Asserter

The Achiever

The Romantic

Moving Around Within the Enneagram

Following the lines in the diagram, the Two moves toward Four in one direction and toward Eight in the other. Twos move toward the positive side of Four when they feel secure; they can also consciously cultivate these positive qualities. Twos move toward the negative side of Eight when in stress; they can consciously try to avoid these negative traits. Read the chapters about types Four and Eight to learn more about them.

When Twos Move Toward the Positive Side of Four They

- admit and accept their painful feelings, including anger, sadness, and loneliness
- express themselves more creatively and artistically; explore their inner world

- express their own needs more, including saying no
- find other sources of self-worth besides helping
- learn to be alone and become more contemplative

When Twos Move Toward the Negative Side of Four They

- compare themselves with others, lament, and feel envious
- become more self-absorbed, withdrawn, and depressed

When Twos Move Toward the Negative Side of Eight They

- stop being kind and loving; become irritable and attack sharply
- become hardened, distrustful, and isolated
- blame and make demands
- become controlling: try to take charge of everyone and everything

When Twos Move Toward the Positive Side of Eight They

- feel more self-confident and powerful
- become more honest and straightforward
- become less concerned with others' opinions of them

Practical Suggestions and Exercises for a Two

1. Self-Esteem

- Engage in some activities that give you pleasure and satisfaction but that do not involve being with others.
- Exercise, meditate, and walk alone to bring the focus back to yourself.
- Reparent your inner child by talking to yourself in nurturing and loving ways, as you would to a real child. Stay in the parent stance, however.
- Give yourself some of the attention and pampering that you usually give to others.

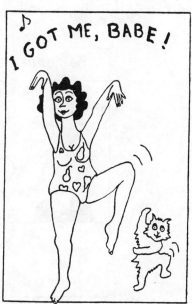

I GOT ME, BABE!

- Go to a counselor regularly to learn how to discuss your own problems.
- Value the love that *is* in your life instead of focusing on what's missing.

2. Assertiveness

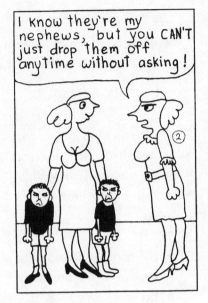

- Set limits. Say, "No, this is not a good time to talk," or "No, I will not be able to help," when you feel that another's request or demand would be too stressful for you.
- Get in touch with your angry feelings. Sometimes Twos feel overwhelmed and cry instead of dealing directly with what made them angry.
- Write down your resentments on a daily basis to become more aware of them.
- If you feel you are being treated unfairly or being taken advantage of, speak up as reasonably as possible, right away.

3. Relationships

- Try to be your own person, not the one others want you to be.
- Refrain from automatically offering help and giving advice; wait until asked.

Be honest about what you want.

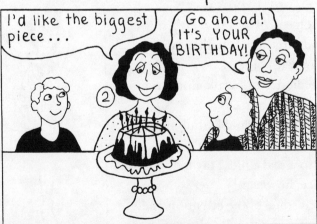

- Take pleasure in giving in little ways. Stop overgiving, and graciously accept when people give to you.

For Parents
- Help your children become independent.
- Learn ways to stop excessive worrying about your grown children. Develop interests of your own to help you detach.
- Beware of the tendency to instill guilt in your children.

4. Codependency
- Go slowly when entering a new relationship. Get information. Be objective.
- Avoid relationships with needy or unavailable people. Only accept friendships and partnerships that are equal.
- Don't rescue people. Allow others to be responsible for their own behavior.
- Be aware that your desire for sex may camouflage your need for attention and approval.
- Resist rushing into another relationship when one ends. Take time to learn why the relationship failed, get to know yourself, and develop other interests.

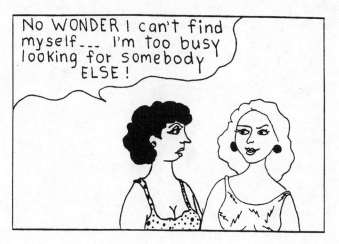

5. Work
- Set limits so you don't take on more than your fair share of work.
- Develop assertiveness and objectivity.

- Find work that is suited to your personality, your interests, and your training.

Things Twos Would Never Dream of Doing

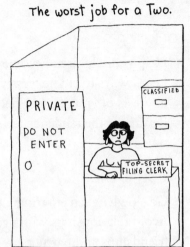

The worst job for a Two.

- refusing to smile at anyone for a month
- accepting all compliments with a simple "thank you" and not discounting them, brushing them off, or explaining why they weren't deserved
- not wanting to take home an adorable kitten they had found
- not wanting to pay friends back tenfold after the friends had done them a favor
- not giving a second thought to a co-worker's snub
- telling a friend they couldn't give them a ride to the airport, and not giving or making up any excuses
- saying only a simple "good-bye" and not adding "good luck," "stay well," or "have a nice day!"

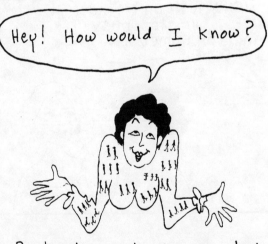

Hey! How would I know?

Pretend you don't know what the solution is to everybody's problem.

Positive Things to Say to Yourself

I am as important as everyone else.

It is as important for me to receive love and help as to give them.

I will speak up for what I want.

I do not have to give to be loved.

It is important for me to spend some quality time by myself.

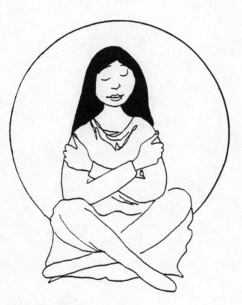

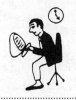

THE

Achiever

Work is more fun than fun.
—Noel Coward

Threes are motivated by the need to be productive, achieve success, and avoid failure.

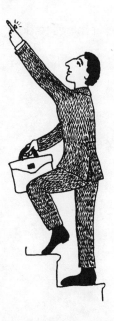

Threes at their BEST are	Threes at their WORST are
optimistic	deceptive
confident	narcissistic
industrious	pretentious
efficient	vain
self-propelled	superficial
energetic	vindictive
practical	overly competitive

Personality Inventory

Check what describes you when you were (or if you are now) under the age of 25.

☐ 1 I'm almost always busy.

☐ 2 I like to make to-do lists, progress charts, and schedules for myself.

☐ 3 I don't mind being asked to work overtime.

☐ 4 I have an optimistic attitude.

☐ 5 I go full force until I get the job done.

☐ 6 I believe in doing things as expediently as possible.

☐ 7 It is important for people to better themselves and live up to their potential.

☐ 8 I'm not interested in talking a lot about my personal life.

☐ 9 I try not to let illness stop me from doing anything.

☐ 10 I hate to see jobs undone.

☐ 11 I tend to put work before other things.

☐ 12 I can't understand people who are bored. I never run out of things to do.

☐ 13 It is sometimes difficult for me to get in touch with my feelings.

☐ 14 I work very hard to take care of and provide for my family.

☐ 15 I like identifying with competent groups or important people.

☐ 16 I try to present myself well and make a good first impression.

☐ 17 Financial security is extremely important to me.

☐ 18 I generally feel pretty good about myself.

☐ 19 People often look to me to run the show.

☐ 20 I like to stand out in some way.

achiever (3)

How to Get Along with Me

- Leave me alone when I am doing my work.
- Give me honest, but not unduly critical or judgmental, feedback.
- Help me keep my environment harmonious and peaceful.
- Don't burden me with negative emotions.
- Tell me you like being around me.
- Tell me when you're proud of me or my accomplishments.

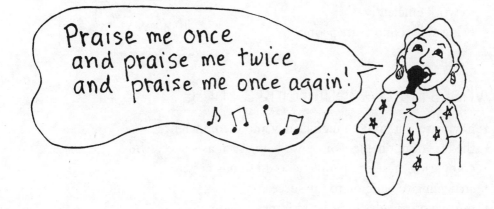

Relationships

Threes at their best in a relationship value and accept their partners. They are playful, giving, responsible, and well regarded by others in the community.

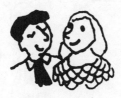

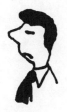

Threes at their worst in a relationship are pre-occupied with work and projects. They are self-absorbed, defensive, impatient, dishonest, and controlling.

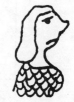

41

What I Like About Being a Three

- being optimistic, friendly, and upbeat
- providing well for my family
- being able to recover quickly from setbacks and to charge ahead to the next challenge
- staying informed, knowing what's going on
- being competent and able to get things to work efficiently
- being able to motivate people

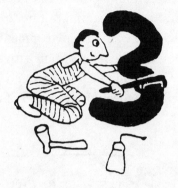

What's Hard About Being a Three

- having to put up with inefficiency and incompetence
- the fear of not being—or of not being seen as—successful
- comparing myself to people who do things better
- struggling to hang on to my success
- putting on facades in order to impress people
- always being "on." It's exhausting.

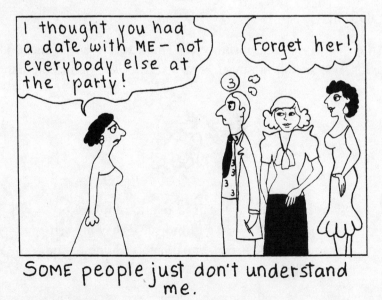

Typical Thoughts of a Three

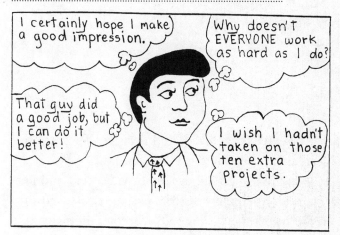

I certainly hope I make a good impression.

Why doesn't EVERYONE work as hard as I do?

That guy did a good job, but I can do it better!

I wish I hadn't taken on those ten extra projects.

Threes as Children Often

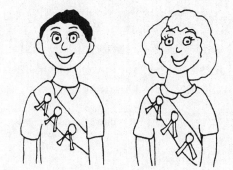

- work hard to receive appreciation for their accomplishments
- are well liked by other children and by adults
- are among the most capable and responsible children in their class or school
- are active in school government and clubs or are quietly busy working on their own projects

Threes as Parents

- are consistent, dependable, and loyal
- struggle between wanting to spend time with their children and wanting to get more work done
- expect their children to be responsible and organized

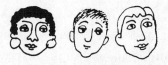

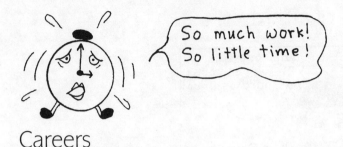

Careers

Threes are hardworking, goal oriented, organized, and decisive. They are frequently in management or leadership positions in business, law, banking, the computer field, and politics. Being in the public eye, as broadcasters and performers, is also common. The more helping-oriented Threes tend to go into teaching, social services, or the health field. They also become homemakers who put tremendous energy into their responsibilities.

And Free Time (If Any)

Many Threes enjoy socializing or doing volunteer work for charities and political campaigns. Some are more likely to spend free time working on hobbies and projects. Most Threes like to exercise and stay in good shape.

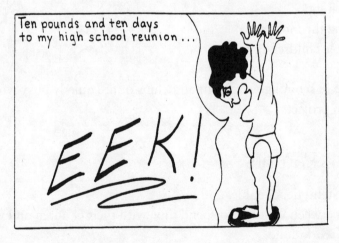

Comments About Threes

"She writes the clearest and most concise reports in my company and inspires us with her work habits, enthusiasm, and sunny disposition."

"He is charming and has a way of making everyone feel special and important."

"My friend is self-assured and confident, has a lot of drive, and does more in a day than most people can do in a week."

"She is the most focused and purposeful person I know. She has made such great improvements in our community that I hope she runs for president."

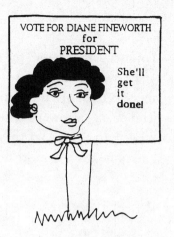

Wings

Your personality may blend into or be influenced by the types on either side of yours. A strong wing can make a big difference in your personality.

Threes with a more developed Two wing tend to be warmer, more encouraging, sociable, popular, and seductive.

Threes with a more developed Four wing tend to be more introspective, sensitive, artistic, imaginative, and pretentious.

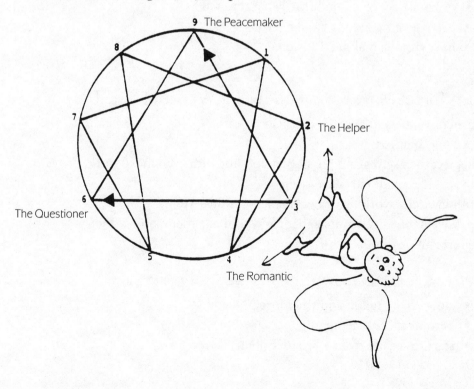

Moving Around Within the Enneagram

Following the lines in the diagram, the Three moves toward Six in one direction and toward Nine in the other. Threes move toward the positive side of Six when they feel secure; they can also consciously cultivate these positive qualities. Threes move toward the negative side of Nine when in stress; they can consciously try to avoid these negative traits. Read the chapters about types Six and Nine to learn more about them.

When Threes Move Toward the Positive Side of Six They

- spend more time with, and become more committed to, family and friends
- value what's best for the group
- get more in touch with their feelings
- become more vulnerable

When Threes Move Toward the Negative Side of Six They

- become dependent and fear being rejected
- become more anxious and nervous
- have trouble making decisions

When Threes Move Toward the Negative Side of Nine They

- procrastinate and become indecisive
- become apathetic
- neglect themselves and possibly numb out with even more work, drugs, food, alcohol, or excessive sleep
- run in circles working or become less productive
- passive-aggressively punish people who make them look at their shortcomings

When Threes Move Toward the Positive Side of Nine They

- slow down, relax, and feel more peaceful
- become more receptive
- start to see life from a broader point of view

Practical Suggestions and Exercises for a Three

1. Relaxation and Self-Nurturing

The hardest work is to go idle.

—Jewish proverb

- Since the stress of overworking can lead to physical and emotional problems, schedule time every day to rest, and practice meditation or stress-reduction techniques. Include massages, steam baths, or saunas.
- Make time for doing some of the activities you value aside from work.
- Reduce stress by appreciating and accepting your present level of success.
- Try to become more aware of your real desires and preferences.
- Take a vacation and leave all your work at home.

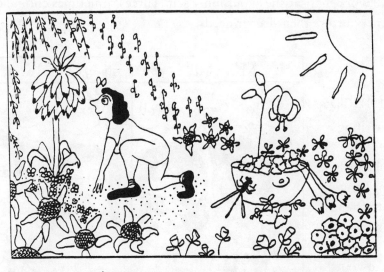

Take time to smell the flowers.

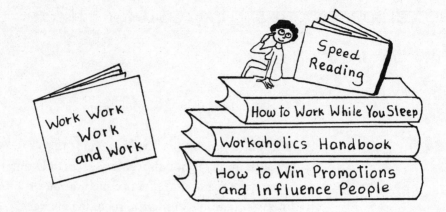

2. Work

- Realize others are probably not as efficient as you are. Many people do not have your energy or ability to focus.
- Beware of the negative impact that forging ahead on your own can have on others. Have other work available to do while you wait.
- Make a special effort to show appreciation and acknowledge others' contributions.
- Beware of being overly hasty in making decisions; take time to factor in all sides, including the human element.
- Explore work that satisfies your inner self. Threes sometimes choose careers that don't nurture their deeper needs.

3. Relationships

- When writing your weekly schedule, include time for hanging out with friends and family.
- When a loved one comes to you with a problem,

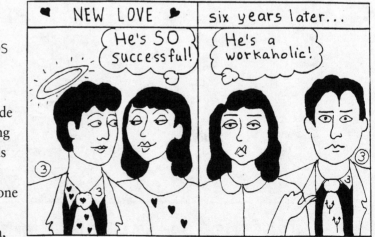

listen without giving advice unless it is asked for. He or she may be in need of a sympathetic ear.

- Remember to express appreciation to your partner. Some Threes think they are the more important one of the couple because they accomplish so much.

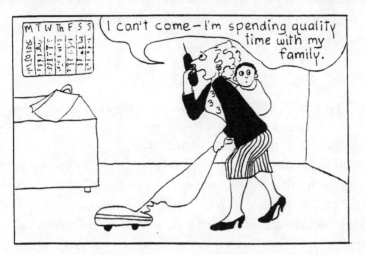

- Do volunteer work, where you give to others purely for the sake of giving.
- Search for the grain of truth in people's criticisms of you.
- Try to stick to who you really are. Threes sometimes try to win people over by changing colors like a chameleon, which backfires when relationships deepen.
- Notice undesirable traits about yourself, for instance, "I do not pay attention to my partner when she needs to talk, but I expect her to give me her full attention when I talk."

For Parents

- Be aware of your high expectations. Excessive pressure on your children will create emotional problems for them.

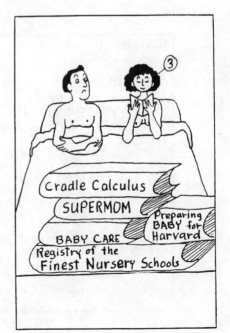

4. Feelings

- Become aware of the difference between your real feelings and feelings you "put on" because they seem appropriate for the occasion.
- Notice the habit of jumping into activity when anxiety begins to arise.
- Allow yourself to be vulnerable: express your hurt and disappointment.

Things Threes Would Never Dream of Doing

- not making a list of goals for an entire week
- saying nothing about their accomplishments at their high school reunion
- refraining from using the "seductive-eye technique" on the person they are interested in
- not taking over the meeting when it is being run inefficiently or ineffectively
- seeing a job that needs doing and not making a note of it
- spending one week just sitting at a silent meditation retreat

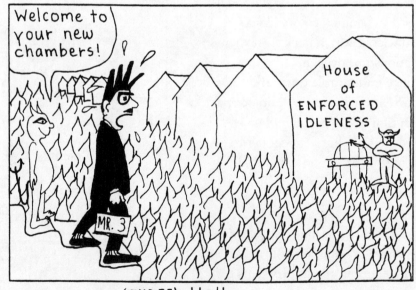

'THREE' Hell

Positive Things to Say to Yourself

My feelings are at least as valuable as my accomplishments.

The most profitable work I can do is to take time to relax and to grow.

I measure my worth by my own standards.

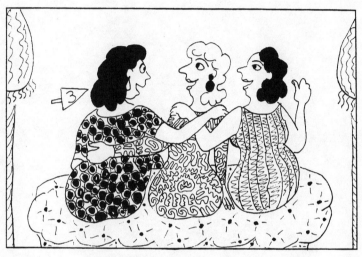

I am loved for who I am —
not for what I do.

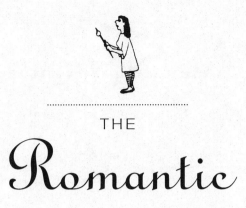

THE

Romantic

*I can stand almost anything
except a succession of ordinary days.*
—Goethe

Fours are motivated by the need to experience their feelings and to be understood, to search for the meaning of life, and to avoid being ordinary.

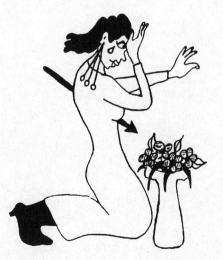

Fours at their BEST are	Fours at their WORST are
warm	depressed
compassionate	self-conscious
introspective	guilt-ridden
expressive	moralistic
creative	withdrawn
intuitive	stubborn
supportive	moody
refined	self-absorbed

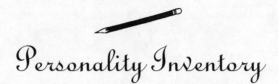

Personality Inventory

Check what describes you when you were (or if you are now) under the age of 25.

- [ ] 1   Being understood is very important to me.
- [ ] 2   My friends say they enjoy my warmth and my different way of looking at life.
- [ ] 3   I can become nonfunctional for hours, days, or weeks when I'm depressed.
- [ ] 4   I am very sensitive to critical remarks and feel hurt at the tiniest slight.
- [ ] 5   It really affects me emotionally when I read upsetting stories in the newspaper.
- [ ] 6   My ideals are very important to me.
- [ ] 7   I cry easily. Beauty, love, sorrow, and pain really touch me.
- [ ] 8   My melancholy moods are real and important. I don't necessarily want to get out of them.
- [ ] 9   I often long for what others have.
- [ ] 10   I try to support my friends, especially when they are in crisis.
- [ ] 11   I live in the past and in the future more than in present-day reality.
- [ ] 12   I place great importance on my intuition.
- [ ] 13   I try to control people at times.
- [ ] 14   I hate insincerity and lack of integrity in others.
- [ ] 15   I have spent years longing for the great love of my life to come along.
- [ ] 16   I focus on what is wrong with me rather than on what is right.
- [ ] 17   I like to be seen as one of a kind.
- [ ] 18   I am always searching for my true self.
- [ ] 19   Sometimes I feel very uncomfortable and different, like an isolated outsider, even when I'm with my friends.
- [ ] 20   When people tell me what to do, I often become rebellious and do, or wish I could do, the opposite.

10
Romantic (4)

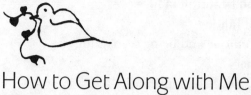

How to Get Along with Me

- Give me plenty of compliments. They mean a lot to me.
- Be a supportive friend or partner. Help me to learn to love and value myself.
- Respect me for my special gifts of intuition and vision.
- Though I don't always want to be cheered up when I'm feeling melancholy, I sometimes like to have someone lighten me up a little.
- Don't tell me I'm too sensitive or that I'm overreacting!

Relationships

Fours at their best in a relationship are empathic, supportive, gentle, playful, passionate, and witty. They are self-revealing and bond easily.

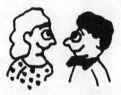

 Fours at their worst in a relationship are too self-absorbed, jealous, emotionally needy, moody, self-righteous, and overly critical. They become hurt and feel rejected easily.

What I Like About Being a Four

- my ability to find meaning in life and to experience feelings at a deep level
- my ability to establish warm connections with people

- admiring what is noble, truthful, and beautiful in life
- my creativity, intuition, and sense of humor
- being unique and being seen as unique by others
- having aesthetic sensibilities
- being able to easily pick up the feelings of people around me

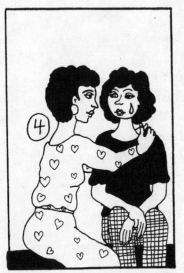

being supportive of my friends

What's Hard About Being a Four

- experiencing dark moods of emptiness and despair
- feelings of self-hatred and shame; believing I don't deserve to be loved
- feeling guilty when I disappoint people
- feeling hurt or attacked when someone misunderstands me
- expecting too much from myself and life
- fearing being abandoned
- obsessing over resentments
- longing for what I don't have

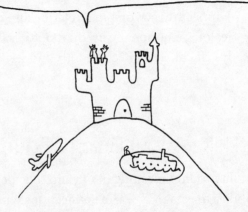

Three Oscars, the Pulitzer Prize — my Prince Charming and wonderful kids — ten pots of gold.... but something is STILL missing!

Typical Thoughts of a Four

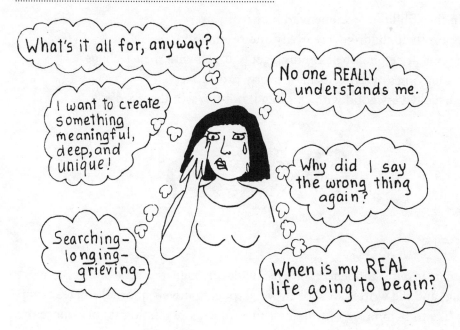

What's it all for, anyway?

No one REALLY understands me.

I want to create something meaningful, deep, and unique!

Why did I say the wrong thing again?

Searching— longing— grieving—

When is my REAL life going to begin?

Fours as Children Often

- have active imaginations: play creatively alone or organize playmates in original games
- are very sensitive
- feel that they don't fit in
- believe they are missing something that other people have
- attach themselves to idealized teachers, heroes, artists, etc.
- become antiauthoritarian or rebellious when criticized or not understood
- feel lonely or abandoned (perhaps as a result of a death or their parents' divorce)

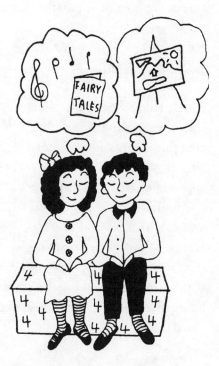

Fours as Parents

- help their children become who they really are
- support their children's creativity and originality
- are good at helping their children get in touch with their feelings
- are sometimes overly critical or overly protective
- are usually very good with children if not too self-absorbed

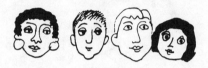

Careers

Fours can inspire, influence, and persuade through the arts (music, fine art, dancing) and the written or spoken word (poetry, novels, journalism, teaching). Many like to help bring out the best in people as psychologists or counselors. Some take pride in the small businesses they own. Often Fours accept mundane jobs to support their creative pursuits.

And Free Time

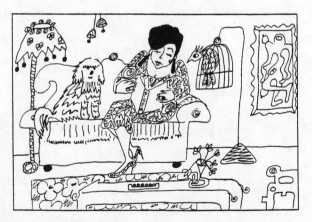

Fours enjoy spending time with their partners and children and maintaining important close friendships. They appreciate nature, pursue spiritual interests, and attend musical, artistic, and literary events. Many enjoy browsing in bookstores, shopping in boutiques, and looking for interesting clothing or one-of-a-kind treasures. Fours often express themselves creatively. Some are active in antiviolence or political causes.

Comments About Fours

"He has a very deep soul. I value him for being my wittiest and most insightful and intellectually stimulating friend."

"The Fours I know have an interesting mixture of qualities: intensity, depth, spirituality, and rebelliousness."

"He runs a very successful business due to his perseverance, determination, and originality."

"She has her own innovative day-care center. She is committed to making it a healthy and creative environment for the children."

"She's a real character. She can usually be found inventing new recipes, floating gardenias in her bathtub, or giving crazy parties."

One should either be a work of art or wear a work of art.

—Oscar Wilde

Wings

Your personality may blend into or be influenced by the types on either side of yours. A strong wing can make a big difference in your personality.

Fours with a Three wing tend to be more extroverted, upbeat, ambitious, flamboyant, and image-conscious.

Fours with a Five wing tend to be more introverted, intellectual, idiosyncratic, reserved, and depressed.

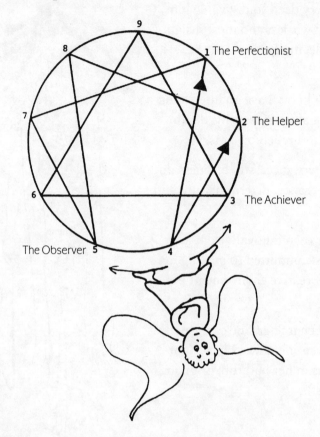

Moving Around Within the Enneagram

Following the lines in the diagram, the Four moves toward One in one direction and toward Two in the other. Fours move toward the positive side of One when they feel secure; they can also consciously cultivate these positive qualities. Fours move toward the negative side of Two when in stress; they can consciously try to avoid these negative traits. Read the chapters about types One and Two to learn more about them.

When Fours Move Toward the Positive Side of One They

- become more self-disciplined and grounded in the here and now
- do more problem solving and become more practical

- shift to accentuating more of the positive and less of the negative
- act on their strong ideals and principles
- become less controlled by their feelings

When Fours Move Toward the Negative Side of One They

- feel critical, judgmental, and angry that no one does anything right
- moralize and preach at people
- feel guilty for not living up to their own expectations

When Fours Move Toward the Negative Side of Two They

- try to manipulate others into loving them in the mistaken belief that another's love will replace their own emptiness and loneliness
- deny and repress their own needs
- become overly dependent
- possibly become ill to get attention or to be special

When Fours Move Toward the Positive Side of Two They

- connect with people in meaningful ways
- become less self-absorbed
- meet others' needs with healthy detachment

Practical Suggestions and Exercises for a Four

1. Self-Esteem

- Be proud of all your special gifts, talents, and accomplishments.
- Work toward fulfilling the needs that were not met in your childhood. Treat yourself lovingly and compassionately.
- Devote yourself to the task of self-discipline.
- Value living in the present.
- Find ways to make everyday duties and responsibilities creative or playful.
- Commit yourself to creative work that will bring out the best in you. Try to make this your source of financial support.
- If it is not possible to make a career of your creativity, make sure you take the time you need for your ideas to germinate in your off-work hours.

- Notice what qualities you admire or envy in others and develop them in yourself.

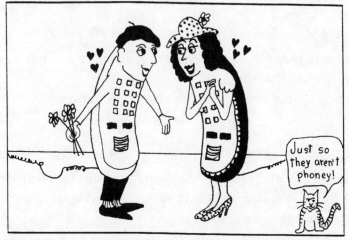

Develop connections with people who have a lot in common with you.

2. Relationships

- Be direct and specific about stating what you want and don't want.
- Be careful not to blow what others say out of proportion. If you feel offended, check to find out what was really meant.
- Develop a strong support system of friends, rather than relying on only one to meet all your emotional needs.
- Deal with interpersonal issues quickly instead of withdrawing from them. Try to be objective and not overpower people with your emotions.

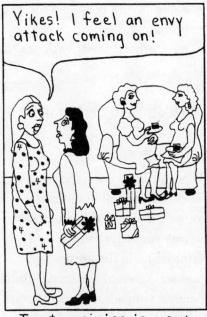

Try to rejoice in your friends' good fortune.

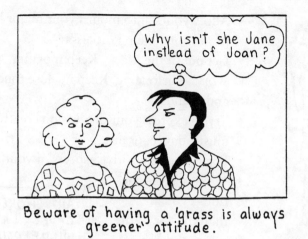

Beware of having a 'grass is always greener' attitude.

3. Feelings and Emotions

- Write your feelings down in the strongest language possible in a letter *that you do not mail.*

- When you have trouble controlling an emotional reaction:

  1. become a detached observer
  2. visualize yourself gradually turning the dial down
  3. stand still and hurt. Remember, it *will* pass.

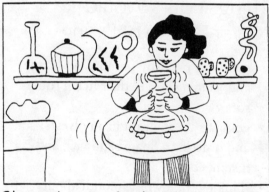

Channel your feelings into creative activities.

This will help you not to be run entirely by your feelings.

- Fours often amplify their feelings out of proportion. See if you are more attached to the intensity of the feeling than to the feeling itself.

4. Avoiding Depression

- As reasonably as possible, confront people who upset you so your anger doesn't turn inward.
- Develop good habits of sleep, exercise, eating, and work.

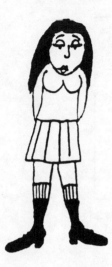

- Allow yourself to mourn your major losses. Get professional help if necessary.
- Get out of the house. Keep moving.
- Work at belonging. Keep in close touch with relatives and friends.
- Try to express your depression creatively: in poetry, music, dance, or art.
- Focus on the positive aspects of your life.
- Make a list of the things you are thankful for. Write it big, and post it on the wall.

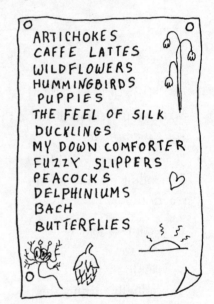

ARTICHOKES
CAFFE LATTES
WILDFLOWERS
HUMMINGBIRDS
PUPPIES
THE FEEL OF SILK
DUCKLINGS
MY DOWN COMFORTER
FUZZY SLIPPERS
PEACOCKS
DELPHINIUMS
BACH
BUTTERFLIES

Things Fours Would Never Dream of Doing

- making a paint-by-number landscape and hanging it over their living room sofa
- going to a restaurant in a polyester suit and ordering a Spam sandwich and instant coffee
- thinking for a whole month about nothing but positive things that have happened in their lives
- deciding that mauve, champagne, and indigo are stupid colors and decorating their house in Happy Pink and Laughing Yellow instead
- deciding that soul-searching is too trite and giving it up
- throwing away old photos of boyfriends or girlfriends *dispassionately*

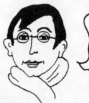

I always forget about it IMMEDIATELY whenever anyone hurts my feelings... like Nancy did on Thursday, August 8, 1989, at 9:37 P.M...

Positive Things to Say to Yourself

I will value each day, no matter how imperfect.

I will relax and enjoy the present.

I am at home in my body, the world, and the universe.
At the heart of my life, all is well.

I am beautiful, capable, and lovable, just as I am.
There is nothing to make up for.

I can be as kind to myself as I am to my best friend.

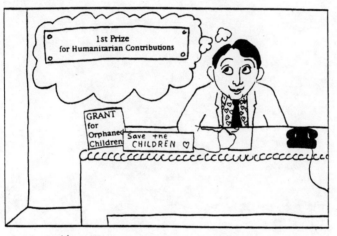

I will make the world a better place
by putting my ideals into action!

COFFEE BREAK

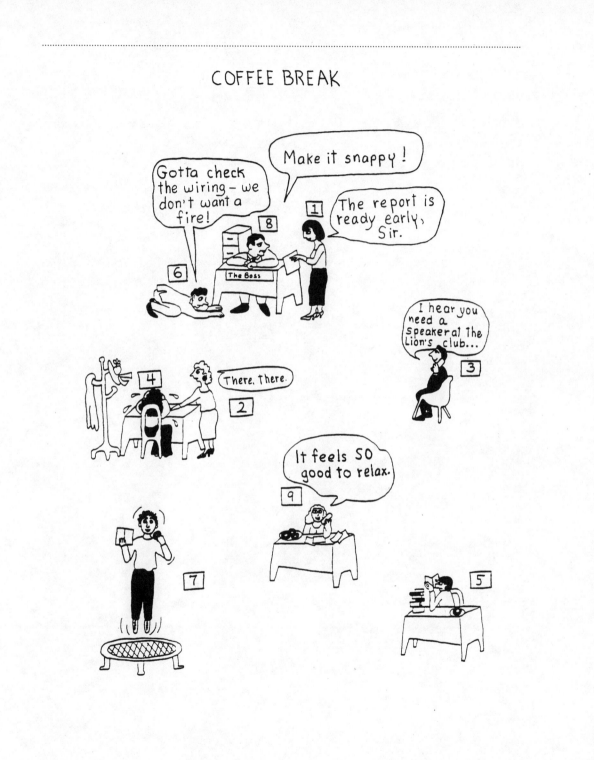

THE

Observer

You can observe a lot just by watching.
—Yogi Berra

Fives are motivated by the need to know and understand everything, to be self-sufficient, and to avoid looking foolish.

Fives at their BEST are	Fives at their WORST are
analytical	intellectually arrogant
persevering	stingy
sensitive	stubborn
wise	distant
objective	critical of others
perceptive	unassertive
self-contained	negative

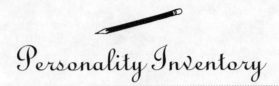

Personality Inventory

Check what describes you when you were (or if you are now) under the age of 25.

☐ 1 I learn from observing or reading as opposed to doing.

☐ 2 It's hard to express my feelings in the moment.

☐ 3 I get lost in my interests and like to be alone with them for hours.

☐ 4 I usually experience my feelings more deeply when I'm by myself.

☐ 5 Sometimes I feel guilty that I'm not generous enough.

☐ 6 I try to conceal my sensitivity to criticism and judgment.

☐ 7 Brash, loud people offend me.

☐ 8 Conforming is distasteful to me.

☐ 9 I like to associate with others who have expertise in my field.

☐ 10 I like having a title (doctor, professor, administrator) to feel proud of.

☐ 11 I have been accused of being negative, cynical, and suspicious.

☐ 12 When I feel socially uncomfortable, I often wish I could disappear.

☐ 13 I am often reluctant to be assertive or aggressive.

☐ 14 I dislike most social events. I'd rather be alone or with a few people I know well.

☐ 15 I sometimes feel shy or awkward.

☐ 16 I get tired when I'm with people for too long.

☐ 17 I feel different from most people.

☐ 18 I feel invisible. It surprises me when anyone notices anything about me.

☐ 19 I don't look for material possessions to make me happy.

☐ 20 Acting calm is a defense. It makes me feel stronger.

13

Observer (5)

How to Get Along with Me

- Be independent, not clingy.
- Speak in a straightforward and brief manner.
- I need time alone to process my feelings and thoughts.
- Remember that if I seem aloof, distant, or arrogant, it *may* be that I am feeling uncomfortable.
- Make me feel welcome, but not too intensely, or I might doubt your sincerity.
- If I become irritated when I have to repeat things, it may be because it was such an effort to get my thoughts out in the first place.
- Don't come on like a bulldozer.
- Help me to avoid my pet peeves: big parties, other people's loud music, overdone emotions, and intrusions on my privacy.

Relationships

Fives at their best in a relationship are kind, perceptive, open-minded, self-sufficient, and trustworthy.

Fives at their worst in a relationship are contentious, suspicious, withdrawn, and negative. They are on their guard against being engulfed.

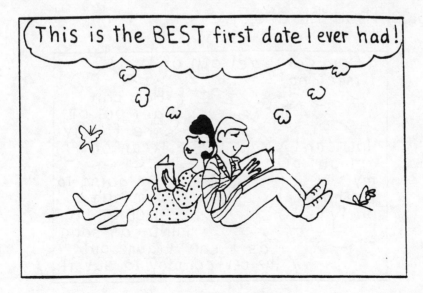

This is the BEST first date I ever had!

What I Like About Being a Five

- standing back and viewing life objectively
- coming to a thorough understanding; perceiving causes and effects
- my sense of integrity: doing what I think is right and not being influenced by social pressure
- not being caught up in material possessions and status
- being calm in a crisis

What's Hard About Being a Five

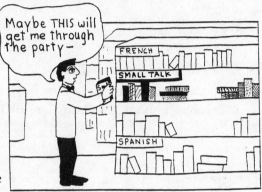

- being slow to put my knowledge and insights out in the world
- feeling bad when I act defensive or like a know-it-all
- being pressured to be with people when I don't want to be
- watching others with better social skills, but less intelligence or technical skill, do better professionally
- having trouble expressing some of my thoughts succinctly

Typical Thoughts of a Five

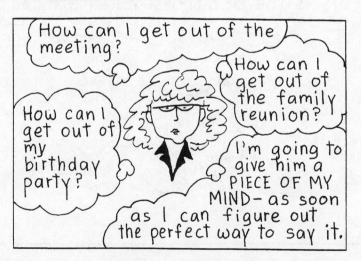

Fives as Children Often

- spend a lot of time alone reading, making collections, and so on
- have a few special friends rather than many
- are very bright and curious and do well in school
- have independent minds and often question their parents and teachers
- watch events from a detached point of view, gathering information
- assume a poker face in order not to look afraid
- are sensitive; avoid interpersonal conflict
- feel intruded upon and controlled and/or ignored and neglected

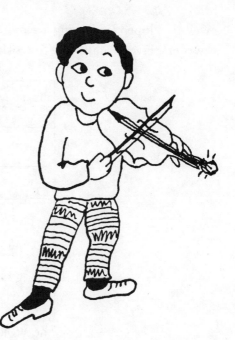

Fives as Parents

- are often kind, perceptive, and devoted
- are sometimes authoritarian and demanding
- may expect more intellectual achievement than is developmentally appropriate
- may be intolerant of their children expressing strong emotions

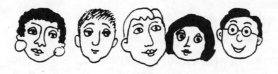

Careers

Fives are often in scientific, technical, or other intellectually demanding fields. They have strong analytical skills and are good at problem solving. Those with a well-developed Four wing are more likely to be counselors, musicians, artists, or writers. Fives usually like to work alone and are independent thinkers.

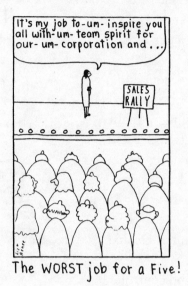

The WORST job for a Five!

And Free Time

Fives enjoy reading books, learning about a subject in depth, having stimulating discussions with friends, going to concerts, museums, and lectures, playing intellectually challenging games, working on their collections or projects, and traveling to study foreign cultures and customs.

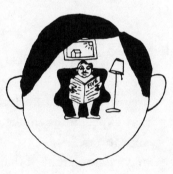

Comments About Fives

"She enjoys her own company. I marvel at the hours she spends by herself reading, gardening, playing music, and analyzing the universe."

"His voice is soft, calm, and soothing. He has a different perspective on things, for example, regarding an insult from someone as an interesting event!"

"She is full of information and innovative ideas. I also like her dry and whimsical sense of humor."

"I was always impressed by how much my Five friend could contribute to any conversation on any subject."

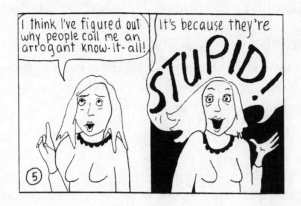

Wings

Your personality may blend into or be influenced by the types on either side of yours. A strong wing can make a big difference in your personality.

Fives with a more developed Four wing tend to be more creative, humanistic, sensitive, empathic, and self-absorbed.

Fives with a more developed Six wing tend to be more loyal, anxious, skeptical, and cautious. They are more likely to be interested in the sciences.

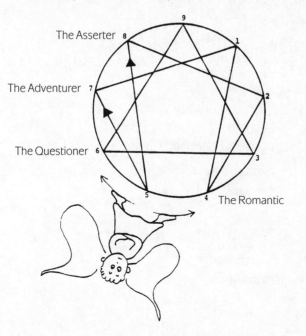

Moving Around Within the Enneagram

Following the lines in the diagram, the Five moves toward Eight in one direction and toward Seven in the other. Fives move toward the positive side of Eight when they feel secure; they can also consciously cultivate these positive qualities. Fives move toward the negative side of Seven when in stress; they can consciously try to avoid these negative traits. Read the chapters about types Eight and Seven to learn more about them.

When Fives Move Toward the Positive Side of Eight They

- get in touch with their body, its power, and its energy by moving away from pure thought and toward action
- trust their instincts more; become more outspoken and spontaneous
- become more assertive, doing whatever it takes to win when they have a justifiable cause to uphold
- become energized and motivated by their anger instead of withdrawing
- defend themselves more effectively; set clear limits

When Fives Move Toward the Negative Side of Eight They

- become punitive
- act unreasonably
- ignore other people's feelings and desires blatantly instead of secretly

When Fives Move Toward the Negative Side of Seven They

- take on new projects impulsively
- become scattered and distracted

When Fives Move Toward the Positive Side of Seven They

- experience life more broadly
- become less self-conscious
- become more fun-loving and uninhibited

Practical Suggestions and Exercises for a Five

1. Getting out of Your Head and into Doing

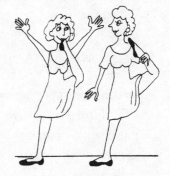

- Take risks and speak up, even if you fear appearing foolish. Emulate some others you know who are not afraid to put their foot in their mouth.
- Become more active by taking up creative or sports activities.
- Value being in the present.
- Go for psychotherapy or body work to learn to express your feelings.

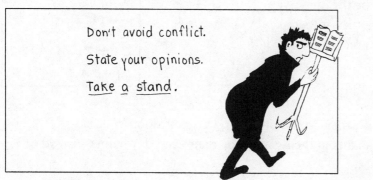

Don't avoid conflict.

State your opinions.

Take a stand.

2. Relationships

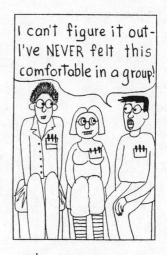

I can't figure it out—I've NEVER felt this comfortable in a group!

- If you have the tendency to deliver long treatises, limit yourself to two or three sentences, then determine if people are interested before continuing. Make it a conversation.
- When you are in a group, be aware of any desperate urge to prove you know something.
- Let others know it when they are important to you.
- When you feel the tendency to give to others, go ahead and do it.
- Ask for what you want, including the setting of limits.

A Nerd-Anon meeting.

- If you desire more experience in interacting with people, become a member of an ongoing therapy group where it is acceptable to speak or not to speak.

Things Fives Would Never Dream of Doing

- missing an opportunity to exhibit their extensive knowledge of an obscure area of their field to their colleagues
- throwing a big party
- volunteering to be the master of ceremonies at their next high school reunion
- subscribing to the newspaper only for the society page

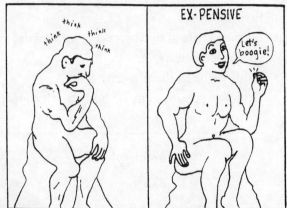

- becoming a used-car salesman or selling vacuums door-to-door
- referring to the plants in their garden by their everyday names instead of their Latin names
- going away with a group where they didn't get a minute to themselves for two weeks

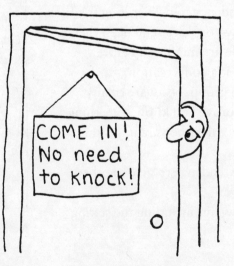

Positive Things to Say to Yourself

Interaction and experience are necessary for real understanding.

I will experience being an individual fully when I empty myself of my preconceived ideas and categories.

I don't have to be the smartest person.

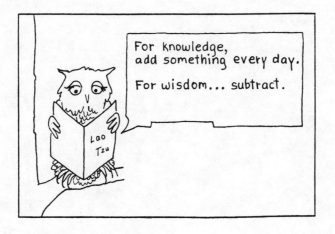

THE

Questioner

I've developed a new philosophy—
I only dread one day at a time.
—Charles M. Schulz

Sixes are motivated by the need for security. Phobic Sixes are outwardly fearful and seek approval. Counterphobic Sixes confront their fear. Both of these aspects can appear in the same person.

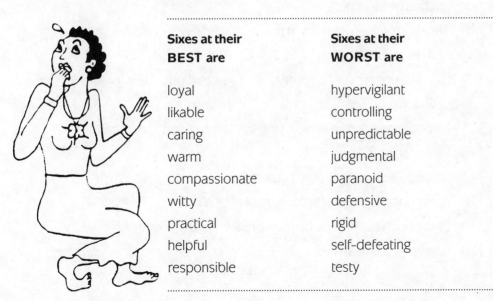

Sixes at their BEST are	Sixes at their WORST are
loyal	hypervigilant
likable	controlling
caring	unpredictable
warm	judgmental
compassionate	paranoid
witty	defensive
practical	rigid
helpful	self-defeating
responsible	testy

Personality Inventory

Check what describes you when you were (or if you are now) under the age of 25.

- ☐ 1 I am nervous around certain authority figures.
- ☐ 2 I am often plagued by doubt.
- ☐ 3 I like to have clear-cut guidelines and to know where I stand.
- ☐ 4 I am always on the alert for danger.
- ☐ 5 I take things too seriously.
- ☐ 6 I constantly question myself about what might go wrong.
- ☐ 7 I often experience criticism as an attack.
- ☐ 8 I often obsess about what my partner is thinking.
- ☐ 9 I can be a very hard worker.
- ☐ 10 My friends think of me as loyal, supportive, and compassionate.
- ☐ 11 I've been told I have a good sense of humor.
- ☐ 12 I follow rules closely (a phobic trait); or I often break rules (a counterphobic trait).
- ☐ 13 The more vulnerable I am in my intimate relationship, the more anxious and testy I become.
- ☐ 14 I tend to either procrastinate or plunge headlong, even into dangerous situations.
- ☐ 15 I am very aware of people trying to manipulate me with flattery.
- ☐ 16 I like predictability.
- ☐ 17 I have sabotaged my own success.
- ☐ 18 I can support people through thick and thin.
- ☐ 19 Being neat and orderly helps me feel more in control of my life.
- ☐ 20 I dislike pretension in people.

3½

Questioner (6)

How to Get Along with Me

- Be direct and clear.
- Listen to me carefully.
- Don't judge me for my anxiety.
- Work things through with me.
- Reassure me that everything is OK between us.
- Laugh and make jokes with me.
- *Gently* push me toward new experiences.
- Try not to overreact to my overreacting.

Let me worry in peace.

Relationships

Sixes at their best in a relationship are warm, playful, open, loyal, supportive, honest, fair, and reliable.

Sixes at their worst in a relationship are suspicious, controlling, inflexible, and sarcastic. They either withdraw or put on a tough act when threatened.

What I Like About Being a Six

- being committed and faithful to family and friends
- being responsible and hardworking
- being compassionate toward others
- having intellect and wit

And What I Like About Being Counterphobic

- being a nonconformist
- confronting danger bravely
- being direct and assertive

What's Hard About Being a Six

- the constant push and pull involved in trying to make up my mind
- procrastinating because of fear of failure; having little confidence in myself
- fearing being abandoned or taken advantage of
- exhausting myself by worrying and scanning for danger

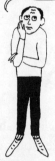

> Today is the day I worried about yesterday.
> Tomorrow is the day I'm worrying about today.
> The next day will be the day ....

- wishing I had a rule book at work so I could do everything right
- being too critical of myself when I haven't lived up to my expectations

Typical Phobic Thoughts of a Six

> Cheer up!
> The worst is yet to come.

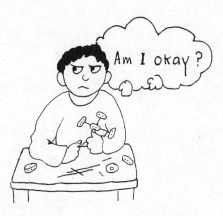

Sixes as Children Often

- are friendly, likable, and dependable, and/or sarcastic, bossy, and stubborn
- are anxious and hypervigilant; anticipate danger
- form a team of "us against them" with a best friend or parent
- look to groups or authorities to protect them and/or question authority and rebel
- are neglected or abused, come from unpredictable or alcoholic families, and/or take on the fearfulness of an overly anxious parent

Sixes as Parents

- are often loving, nurturing, and have a strong sense of duty
- are sometimes reluctant to give their children independence
- worry more than most that their children will get hurt
- sometimes have trouble saying no and setting boundaries

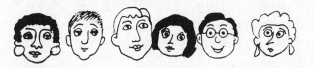

Careers

Though Sixes can be found in almost any career, they are often attracted to the justice system, the military, the corporate world, and academia. Sixes often like being part of a team. Many are in health care and education.

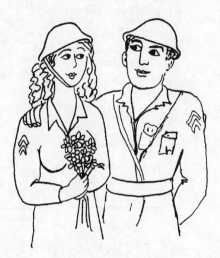

Counterphobic Sixes sometimes have jobs that involve risk. Those who lean toward the antiauthoritarian side are usually happier when self-employed.

If Sixes are unhappy with their work situation, they are likely to become rebellious or secretive.

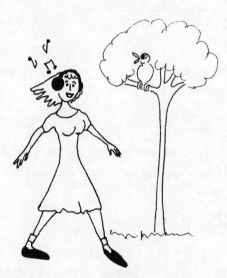

And Free Time

Sixes have a lot of energy and are often very busy. Besides doing the same kinds of leisure activities that the other eight types do, Sixes often enjoy physical exercise and nature. Some belong to groups that help the underdog. Sixes who lean toward the counterphobic frequently engage in dangerous activities or join rebellious groups.

Comments About Sixes

"Lieutenant Holmes never misses a thing! He's been responsible for solving more crimes than anyone else in the department."

"He is the most reliable, trustworthy, and hardworking manager my company has ever had. And he keeps morale high with his terrific sense of humor."

"She was a great teacher. Her warmth and insight inspired me to work hard and get into a good college."

"She's an intelligent, loyal, and lovable friend and has never failed to keep her word or to give me support when I needed it."

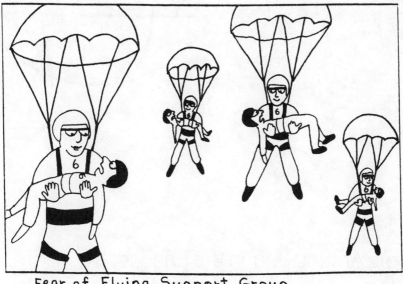

Fear of Flying Support Group

Wings

Your personality may blend into or be influenced by the types on either side of yours. A strong wing can make a big difference in your personality.

Sixes with a more developed Five wing tend to be more introverted, intellectual, cautious, and standoffish.

Sixes with a more developed Seven wing tend to be more extroverted, materialistic, active, and impulsive.

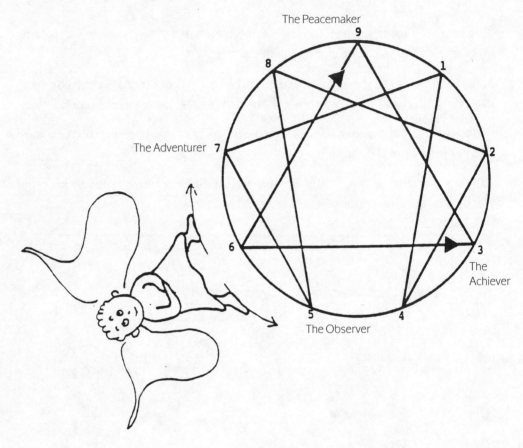

Moving Around Within the Enneagram

Following the lines in the diagram, the Six moves toward Nine in one direction and toward Three in the other. Sixes move toward the positive side of Nine when they feel secure; they can also consciously cultivate these positive qualities. Sixes move toward the negative side of Three when in stress; they can consciously try to avoid these negative traits. Read the chapters about types Nine and Three to learn more about them.

When Sixes Move Toward the Positive Side of Nine They

- empathize more with others
- see things from a broader point of view
- take life less seriously and free up their energy
- put more trust in their own inner authority

When Sixes Move Toward the Negative Side of Nine They

- numb themselves with drugs, television, reading, food, or sleep in order to stop obsessing
- become spaced out and apathetic

When Sixes Move Toward the Negative Side of Three They

- avoid feeling anxious by always being busy; may become workaholics
- become reluctant to try anything new if there is any possibility of failing
- take on a role or image in order to feel more secure
- tell lies about themselves in order to cover up or get ahead

When Sixes Move Toward the Positive Side of Three They

- take decisive and effective action
- feel good about all they accomplish

Practical Suggestions and Exercises for a Six

1. Self-Confidence

- Try to be around people who are accepting, trustworthy, and encouraging.
- Really notice and try to believe the positive things that people say about you.

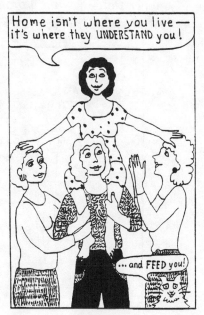

Home isn't where you live — it's where they UNDERSTAND you!

... and FEED you!

- Keep in mind that you *can* change and overcome your fears and learn to take action in the presence of fear.
- Remember that there is no one "right" way to live, as long as you are satisfied inside with what you are doing.
- Pat yourself on the back. Don't wait for someone else to tell you that you did well.
- Write and talk to yourself in nurturing and caring ways.
- Remember it is OK to make mistakes.

2. Relationships

*I always prefer to believe
the best of everybody—
it saves so much trouble.*

—Rudyard Kipling

- Sixes are likely to overreact when they are stressed. Don't underestimate the negative effect this can have on people.
- Give only when you really want to or you will feel drained.
- Reality check with other people: "Were you just thinking . . . ?" or "Were you just thinking what I *thought* you were thinking?"
- Learn to have a sense of humor about your hypervigilance.

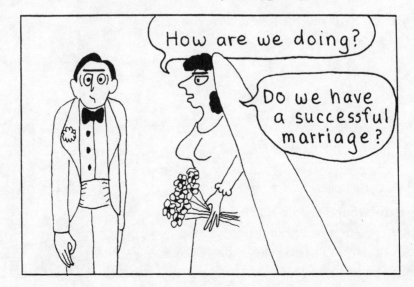

3. Work

- Acknowledge yourself for being a hard worker. Focus on your strengths.
- Break jobs into small parts and do them one at a time.
- If you feel overworked or overstressed because you have taken on too much work, delegate as much as you can to others.
- Be patient when others move at their own pace rather than at yours.

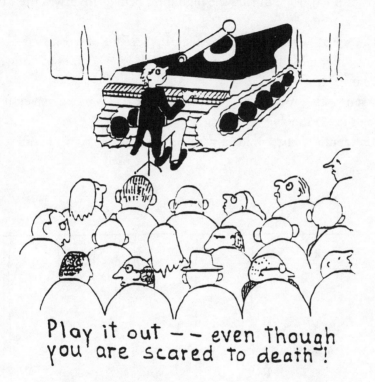

Play it out -- even though you are scared to death!

4. Anxiety and Fear

- Observe your fears without judging yourself for having them.
- Check the facts when anxious. For instance, look up the statistics of the number of plane crashes in a year.
- Learn to accept being in limbo. Your indecisiveness will not last forever.
- Take up meditation, breathing, and visualization techniques, or take a stress-reduction class.
- Visualize a peaceful scene. When a worry creeps in, take deep breaths as you go back to the scene. Practice this regularly.

- Don't call yourself lazy when you are relaxing.
- Take up physical activities: sports, working out, walking.

Things Sixes Would Never Dream of Doing

- hearing a familiar noise during the night and being sure it was the cat and not a burglar
- forgiving themselves after breaking their best friend's favorite vase
- not taking an opinion poll among their friends when contemplating a career change
- going to a new therapist or doctor and not asking even one question about their credentials
- being confident they had made a wise choice after making a major purchase

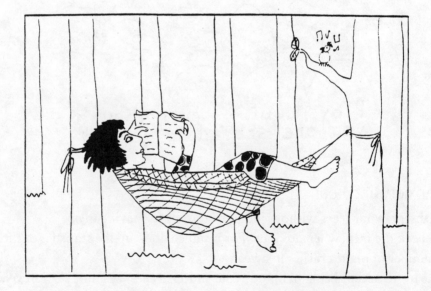

Hortense has no feeling of doom concerning her lost job or her biological clock running out.

Positive Things to Say to Yourself

Being prepared means trusting whatever each moment brings.

I am strong. I am calm. I can do this.

I am OK today, I'll be OK tomorrow.

I am learning to trust my own decisions.

It is OK to take risks and make mistakes.

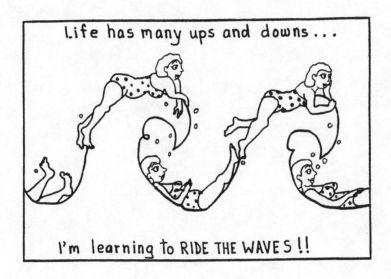

THE

Adventurer

You only live once—
but if you work it right, once is enough.
—Joe E. Lewis

Sevens are motivated by the need to be happy and plan enjoyable activities, to contribute to the world, and to avoid suffering and pain.

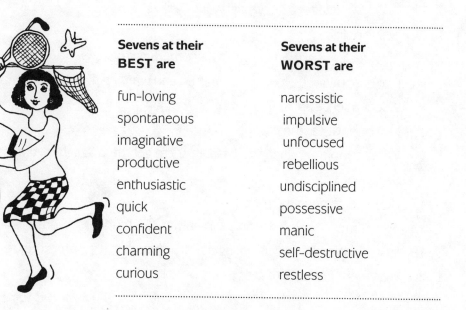

Sevens at their BEST are	Sevens at their WORST are
fun-loving	narcissistic
spontaneous	impulsive
imaginative	unfocused
productive	rebellious
enthusiastic	undisciplined
quick	possessive
confident	manic
charming	self-destructive
curious	restless

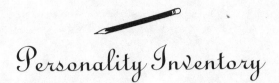

Personality Inventory

Check what describes you when you were (or if you are now) under the age of 25.

- ☐ 1 I enjoy life. I am generally uninhibited and optimistic.
- ☐ 2 I don't like being made to feel obligated or beholden.
- ☐ 3 I am busy and energetic. I seldom get bored if left to do what I want.
- ☐ 4 I often take verbal or physical risks.
- ☐ 5 I usually pick upbeat friends who have similar goals.
- ☐ 6 I'm not an expert in any one thing, but I can do many things well.
- ☐ 7 My style is to go back and forth from one task to another. I like to keep moving.
- ☐ 8 I seem to let go of grievances and recover from loss faster than most people I know.
- ☐ 9 I like myself and I'm good to myself.
- ☐ 10 I like people and they usually like me.
- ☐ 11 I usually manage to get what I want.
- ☐ 12 I value quick wit.
- ☐ 13 I am idealistic. I want to contribute something to the world.
- ☐ 14 I vacillate between feeling committed and wanting my freedom and independence.
- ☐ 15 I am often at ease in groups.
- ☐ 16 When people are unhappy, I usually try to get them to lighten up and see the bright side.
- ☐ 17 I love excitement and travel.
- ☐ 18 Sometimes I feel inferior and sometimes I feel superior to others.
- ☐ 19 I usually say whatever is on my mind. Sometimes it gets me into trouble.
- ☐ 20 I can make great sacrifices to help people.

adventurer (7)

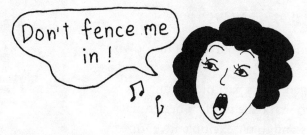

How to Get Along with Me

- Give me companionship, affection, and freedom.
- Engage with me in stimulating conversation and laughter.
- Appreciate my grand visions and listen to my stories.
- Don't try to change my style. Accept me the way I am.
- Be responsible for yourself. I dislike clingy or needy people.
- Don't tell me what to do.

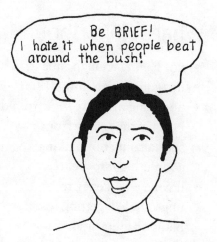

Relationships

Sevens at their best in a relationship are lighthearted, generous, outgoing, caring, and fun. They introduce their friends and loved ones to new activities and adventures.

 Sevens at their worst in a relationship are narcissistic, opinionated, defensive, and distracted. They are often ambivalent about being tied down to a relationship.

What I Like About Being a Seven

- being optimistic and not letting life's troubles get me down
- being spontaneous and free-spirited
- being outspoken and outrageous. It's part of the fun.
- being generous and trying to make the world a better place
- having the guts to take risks and to try exciting adventures
- having such varied interests and abilities

What's Hard About Being a Seven

- not having enough time to do all the things I want
- not completing things I start
- not being able to profit from the benefits that come from specializing; not making a commitment to a career
- having a tendency to be ungrounded; getting lost in plans or fantasies
- feeling confined when I'm in a one-to-one relationship

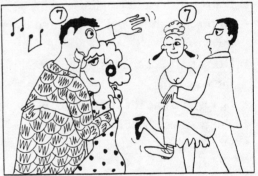

We have to keep our options open!

Typical Thoughts of a Seven

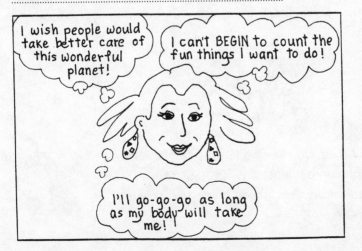

Sevens as Children Often

- are action oriented and adventuresome
- drum up excitement
- prefer being with other children to being alone
- finesse their way around adults
- dream of the freedom they'll have when they grow up

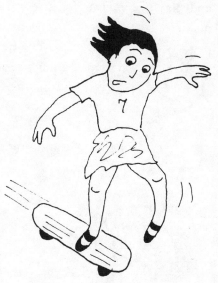

Sevens as Parents

- are often enthusiastic and generous
- want their children to be exposed to many adventures in life
- may be too busy with their own activities to be attentive

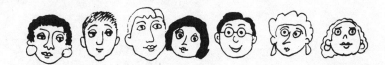

Careers

Many Sevens have several careers at once or jobs where they travel a lot (as pilots, flight attendants, or photographers, for example). Some like using tools or machines or working outdoors. Others prefer solving problems as entrepreneurs or troubleshooters. Still others are in the helping professions as teachers, nurses, or counselors. Sevens are not likely to be found in repetitive work (in assembly lines or accounting, for instance). They like challenges and think quickly in emergencies.

And Free Time

Sevens enjoy traveling, flirting with danger (skydiving, hang gliding, parasailing, rock climbing, driving fast), having interesting

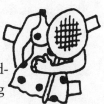

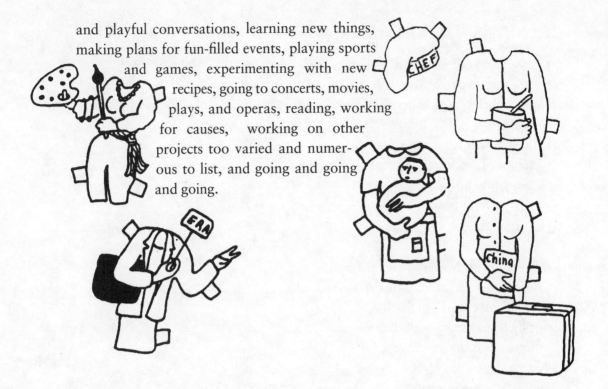

and playful conversations, learning new things, making plans for fun-filled events, playing sports and games, experimenting with new recipes, going to concerts, movies, plays, and operas, reading, working for causes, working on other projects too varied and numerous to list, and going and going and going.

Comments About Sevens

"When I need cheering up, I call my Seven friend and get a dose of her sparkle and optimism. It never fails to work."

"He's hooked on new ideas and possibilities; he's interested in jazz now and has practically every CD there is. Last year he was exploring caves for three months and before that went to cooking school in France."

"Her life is inspiring: She went to Africa, set up a clinic, and saved hundreds of babies. Now she volunteers at the hospital to hold crack babies. On weekends

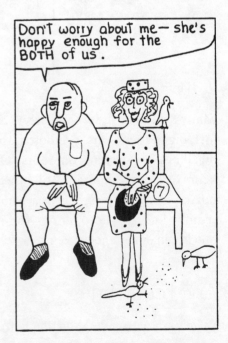

Don't worry about me— she's happy enough for the BOTH of us.

she hikes in the mountains, when she isn't throwing parties or going to the hot springs."

"He was a perfect grandfather! We worked side by side in his workshop for hours. Then we'd go to a baseball game, visit his cronies downtown, and take a ride in the country. At night he'd tell stories about the old gold-mining days. He used to crack me up when he'd take out his false teeth and rattle them at me."

Wings

Your personality may blend into or be influenced by the types on either side of yours. A strong wing can make a big difference in your personality.

Sevens with a more developed Six wing tend to be more loyal, endearing, responsible, and anxious.

Sevens with a more developed Eight wing tend to be more exuberant, aggressive, competitive, and materialistic.

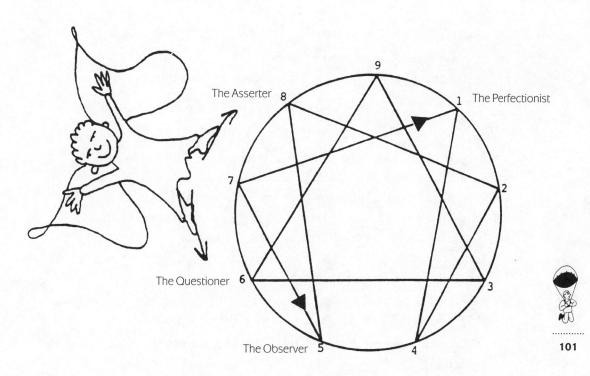

Moving Around Within the Enneagram

Following the lines in the diagram, the Seven moves toward Five in one direction and toward One in the other. Sevens move toward the positive side of Five when they feel secure; they can also consciously cultivate these positive qualities. Sevens move toward the negative side of One when in stress; they can consciously try to avoid these negative traits. Read the chapters about types Five and One to learn more about them.

When Sevens Move Toward the Positive Side of Five They

- become quieter and more introspective and objective
- explore subjects in depth and place more value on wisdom and self-discipline
- become more accepting of both polarities of life: good and bad, happy and sad
- become more serious and are taken more seriously
- get in touch with their fears

When Sevens Move Toward the Negative Side of Five They

- push their theories onto people
- become more self-absorbed and escape responsibilities

When Sevens Move Toward the Negative Side of One They

- become cynical and hypercritical; nitpick, snarl, and try to change people
- become judgmental of themselves and others; can't laugh at themselves
- think in terms of black and white and "know" they have the truth
- blame others for preventing them from having fun
- become obsessive about an idea or project
- feel a pervasive, low-level irritability

When Sevens Move Toward the Positive Side of One They

- become more productive and follow through; put their ideals into action

- become less interested in pleasing themselves and more interested in the welfare of others
- weigh their options more wisely

Practical Suggestions and Exercises for a Seven

1. Health

- Cultivate healthy habits of eating, sleeping, and exercise. Some Sevens have the tendency to go to extremes and neglect their health.
- Take up an exercise program—swimming or tai chi, for example.
- Be careful not to eat, drink, or spend to excess when you are stressed.

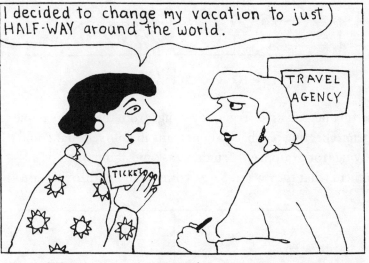

Don't take on more than you can handle.

2. Stress

- Be grateful for what you have instead of focusing on what you want.
- Don't tune out problems, hoping they will go away. Find a friend or counselor to talk with so stress doesn't build.
- Remove your rose-colored glasses and take into account the dark or negative side of life for reality and balance. Realize that positive thinking won't solve every problem.
- Accept feelings, trusting they will pass.

3. Relationships

- In an intimate relationship, how much time you spend together and apart is likely to be a problem. Try to reach agreement about this early on.
- Set aside time for intimacy with your partner.

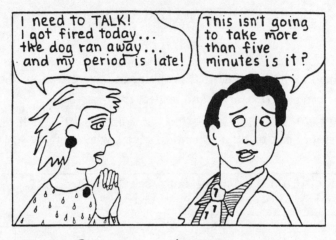

Be a good listener.

- Be tactful and sensitive. Try to see things from the other's point of view.
- Be open to hearing feedback about traits in yourself that could use some improving (for example: "You don't ask me about *my* day").
- Ask others what *they* want. Sevens often don't realize they are self-centered.

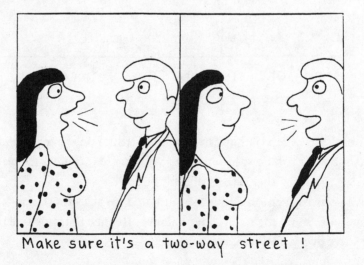

Make sure it's a two-way street !

4. Work

- Consider working for yourself.
- Don't expect others to keep up with your fast pace.
- Concentrate on the work at hand instead of imagining other things you might be doing.
- Remember that hard work will pay off and result in satisfaction. Sevens often feel that if it's not pleasurable, it's not worth doing.
- Find a career where you can put your ideals into action.

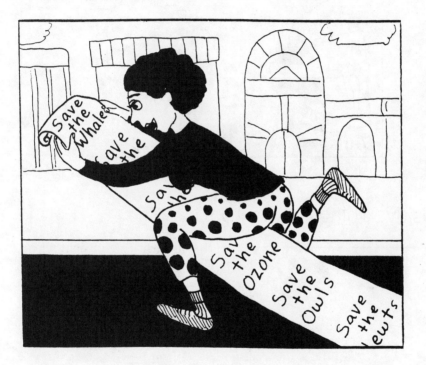

Things Sevens Would Never Dream of Doing

- finishing all the books they were reading before starting a new one
- making to-do lists for the week and following them exactly
- telling stories without exaggerating
- spending six months at a Zen center in silent meditation
- spending a whole day with a friend and not suggesting even one way she or he could do a job faster by taking a few shortcuts

- volunteering to work on a grief hotline
- spending twelve hours listening to a friend unload her problems and talk about herself

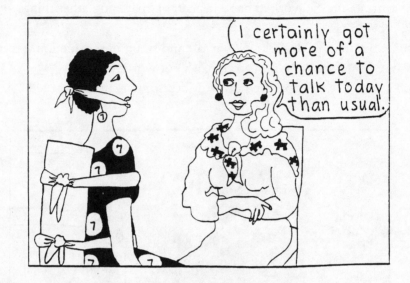

Positive Things to Say to Yourself

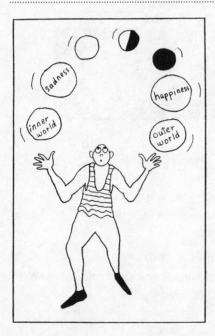

Truth and clarity are in sight when dark is balanced with the light.

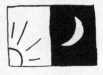

I have enough. There is enough. I need no more.

THE

Asserter

Never go to bed mad—
stay up and fight!

Eights are motivated by the need to be self-reliant and strong and to avoid feeling weak or dependent.

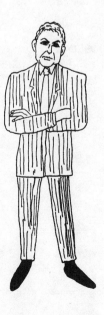

Eights at their BEST are	Eights at their WORST are
direct	controlling
authoritative	rebellious
loyal	insensitive
energetic	domineering
earthy	self-centered
protective	skeptical
self-confident	aggressive

Personality Inventory

Check what describes you when you were (or if you are now) under the age of 25.

- ☐ 1   I can be assertive and aggressive when I need to be.
- ☐ 2   I can't stand being used or manipulated.
- ☐ 3   I value being direct and honest; I put my cards on the table.
- ☐ 4   I am an individualist and a nonconformist.
- ☐ 5   I respect people who stand up for themselves.
- ☐ 6   I will go to any lengths to protect those I love.
- ☐ 7   I fight for what is right.
- ☐ 8   I support the underdog.
- ☐ 9   Making decisions is not difficult for me.
- ☐ 10   Self-reliance and independence are important.
- ☐ 11   I have overindulged in food or drugs.
- ☐ 12   Some people take offense at my bluntness.
- ☐ 13   When I enter a new group, I know immediately who the most powerful person is.
- ☐ 14   I work hard and I know how to get things done.
- ☐ 15   In a group I am sometimes an observer rather than a participant.
- ☐ 16   I like excitement and stimulation.
- ☐ 17   Sometimes I like to spar with people, especially when I feel safe.
- ☐ 18   I am vulnerable and loving when I really trust someone.
- ☐ 19   Overly nice or flattering people bother me.
- ☐ 20   Pretense is particularly distasteful to me.

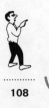

asserter (8)

How to Get Along with Me

- Stand up for yourself . . . and me.
- Be confident, strong, and direct.
- Don't gossip about me or betray my trust.
- Be vulnerable and share your feelings. See and acknowledge my tender, vulnerable side.
- Give me space to be alone.
- Acknowledge the contributions I make, but don't flatter me.
- I often speak in an assertive way. Don't automatically assume it's a personal attack.
- When I scream, curse, and stomp around, try to remember that's just the way I am.

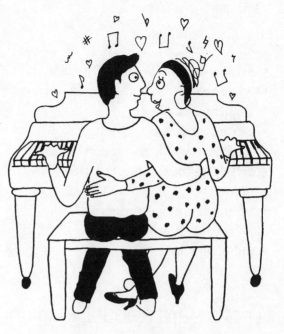

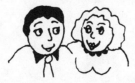

I like the feeling of a close connection.

Relationships

Eights at their best in a relationship are loyal, caring, positive, playful, truthful, straightforward, committed, generous, and supportive.

Eights at their worst in a relationship are demanding, arrogant, combative, possessive, uncompromising, and quick to find fault.

What I Like About Being an Eight

- being independent and self-reliant
- being able to take charge and meet challenges head on
- being courageous, straightforward, and honest
- getting all the enjoyment I can out of life
- supporting, empowering, and protecting those close to me
- upholding just causes

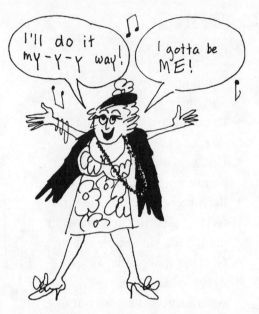

What's Hard About Being an Eight

Women Eights sometimes have a hard time in our society because their strength and boldness are considered "masculine" traits.

- overwhelming people with my bluntness; scaring them away when I don't intend to
- being restless and impatient with others' incompetence
- sticking my neck out for people and receiving no appreciation for it
- never forgetting injuries or injustices
- putting too much pressure on myself
- getting high blood pressure when people don't obey the rules or when things don't go right

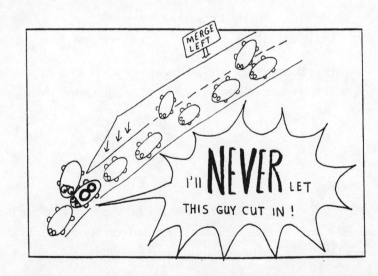

Typical Thoughts of an Eight

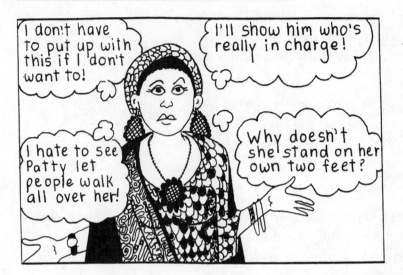

I'd rather be strongly wrong than weakly right.

—Tallulah Bankhead

Eights as Children Often

- are independent; have an inner strength and a fighting spirit
- are sometimes loners
- seize control so they won't *be* controlled
- figure out others' weaknesses
- attack verbally or physically when provoked
- take charge in the family because they perceive themselves as the strongest, or grow up in difficult or abusive surroundings

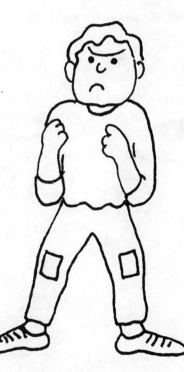

Eights as Parents

- are often loyal, caring, involved, and devoted
- are sometimes overprotective
- can be demanding, controlling, and rigid

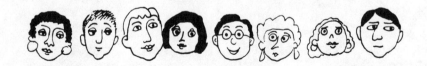

Careers

Eights are good at taking the initiative to move ahead. They want to be in charge. Since they want the freedom to make their own choices, they are often self-employed. Eights have a strong need for financial security. Many are entrepreneurs, business executives, lawyers, military and union leaders, and sports figures. They are also in teaching and the helping and health professions. Eights are attracted to careers in which they can demonstrate their willingness to accept responsibility and take on and resolve difficult problems.

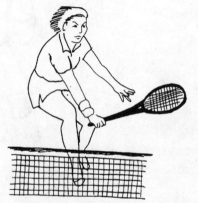

And Free Time

Eights like intellectual and/or physical challenges and often crusade for causes. They are energetic and often enjoy the out-of-doors.

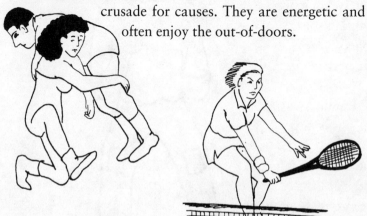

Comments About Eights

"I can be honest and say what is on my mind when I'm with him. In fact, if I'm not frank I feel I've let him down."

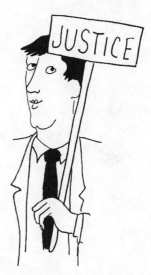

"She is so outrageous! She dresses however she pleases and doesn't care what anyone else thinks. I admire her attitude and her individuality."

"She is vibrant, intense, and earthy. She says things that nobody else has the courage to say, and she inspires me to speak my mind."

"His style of running the company is very practical. He knows how to delegate responsibility, and he always shoots straight from the hip. Because you know exactly what he wants you to do, he is a very effective boss."

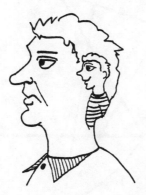

Mike is a powerful guy — yet inside he has a gentle soul.

Wings

Your personality may blend into or be influenced by the types on either side of yours. A strong wing can make a big difference in your personality.

Eights with a more developed Seven wing tend to be more extroverted, enterprising, energetic, quick, and egocentric.

Eights with a more developed Nine wing tend to be more mild-mannered, gentle, receptive, and quietly strong.

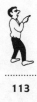

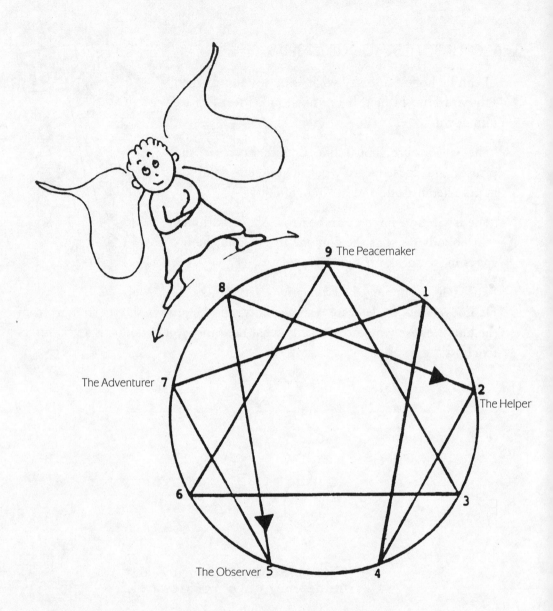

9 The Peacemaker

8

1

The Adventurer 7

2 The Helper

6

3

The Observer 5

4

Moving Around Within the Enneagram

Following the lines in the diagram, the Eight moves toward Two in one direction and toward Five in the other. Eights move toward the positive side of Two when they feel secure; they can also consciously cultivate these positive qualities. Eights move toward the negative side of Five when in stress; they can consciously try to avoid these negative traits. Read the chapters about types Two and Five to learn more about them.

When Eights Move Toward the Positive Side of Two They

- open up to others and reveal their vulnerability
- become more concerned for the welfare of others
- become more loving and lovable; express their soft, gentle, and tender sides

When Eights Move Toward the Negative Side of Two They

- become overly dependent
- place unrealistic demands on others
- become more defensive and overreactive

When Eights Move Toward the Negative Side of Five They

- withdraw and take less action in the world
- become less in touch with their feelings
- fear that others will turn on them
- become defeated and depressed
- may feel guilty and turn their aggression against themselves

When Eights Move Toward the Positive Side of Five They

- step back and see things from a more objective point of view
- think things through more thoroughly before acting

Practical Suggestions and Exercises for an Eight

1. Relationships

- Resist dismissing or invalidating the other's experience or views.
- Beware that when you are "direct" you may unintentionally intimidate others.
- Express your appreciation out loud and often.

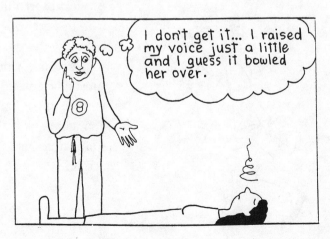

I don't get it... I raised my voice just a little and I guess it bowled her over.

- Avoid driving others as hard as you drive yourself.
- Remember that sparring is stimulating to Eights but not to most other types.
- Learn to negotiate.

No revenge is more honorable than the one not taken.

—Spanish proverb

2. Anger

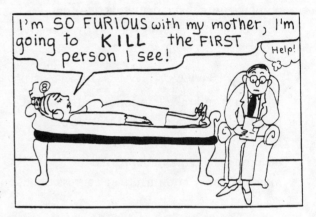

- Eights often become enraged from a previous hurtful comment or action. If you express the hurt quickly and reasonably, it may prevent a later outburst.
- Talk out your anger in therapy or discuss it with a supportive friend.

3. Self-Nurturing

- Find others to have fun with who accept and enjoy your outrageous, nonconforming behavior.

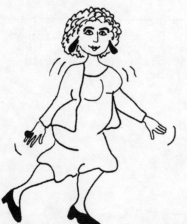

- At work, surround yourself with people who respect your direct approach and are honest with you.
- Join a recovery program if you are a substance abuser.
- Beware of having unrealistic expectations of yourself.
- Make time for enjoyable creative or physical activities.

Things Eights Would Never Dream of Doing

- eliminating all off-color expressions from their vocabulary
- not stating their opinion when they strongly disagree with what is being said
- stepping down as president of the company because they thought someone else could do it better
- playing a tennis match and not trying their hardest to win
- always saying, "Fine, let's do it your way."

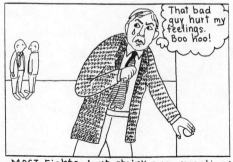

MOST Eights don't shrink away unnoticed when insulted.

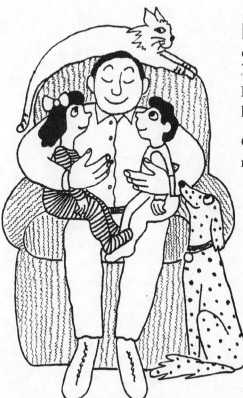

Positive Things to Say to Yourself

I will show my soft and loving side to those I trust.

Good relationships are worth many small compromises.

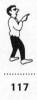

THE

Peacemaker

I always procrastinate when I get around to it.

Nines are motivated by the need to keep the peace, to merge with others, and to avoid conflict. Since they, especially, take on qualities of the other eight types, Nines have many variations in their personalities, from gentle and mild-mannered to independent and forceful.

Nines at their BEST are	Nines at their WORST are
pleasant	spaced-out
peaceful	forgetful
generous	stubborn
patient	obsessive
receptive	apathetic
diplomatic	passive-aggressive
open-minded	judgmental
empathic	unassertive

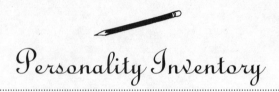

Personality Inventory

Check what describes you when you were (or if you are now) under the age of 25.

- ☐ 1 I often feel in union with nature and people.
- ☐ 2 Making choices can be very difficult. I can see the advantages and disadvantages of every option.
- ☐ 3 It is sometimes hard for me to know what I want when I'm with other people.
- ☐ 4 Others see me as peaceful, but inside I often feel anxious.
- ☐ 5 Instead of tackling what I really need to do, I sometimes do little, unimportant things.
- ☐ 6 When there is unpleasantness going on around me, I just try to think about something else for a while.
- ☐ 7 I usually prefer walking away from a disagreement to confronting someone.
- ☐ 8 If I don't have some routine and structure in my day, I get almost nothing done.
- ☐ 9 I tend to put things off until the last minute, but I almost always get them done.
- ☐ 10 I like to be calm and unhurried, but sometimes I overextend myself.
- ☐ 11 When people try to tell me what to do or try to control me, I get stubborn.
- ☐ 12 I like to be sure to have time in my day for relaxing.
- ☐ 13 Sometimes I feel shy and unsure of myself.
- ☐ 14 I enjoy just hanging out with my partner or friends.
- ☐ 15 Supportive and harmonious relationships are very important to me.
- ☐ 16 I am very sensitive about being judged and take criticism personally.
- ☐ 17 I like to listen and give people support.
- ☐ 18 I focus more on the positive than on the negative.
- ☐ 19 I have trouble getting rid of things.
- ☐ 20 I operate under the principle of inertia: If I'm going, it's easy to keep going, but I sometimes have a hard time getting started.

Peacemaker (9)

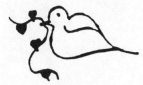

How to Get Along with Me

- If you want me to do something, how you ask is important. I especially don't like expectations or pressure.
- I like to listen and to be of service, but don't take advantage of this.
- Listen until I finish speaking, even though I meander a bit.
- Give me time to finish things and make decisions. It's OK to nudge me gently and nonjudgmentally.
- Ask me questions to help me get clear.
- Tell me when you like how I look. I'm not averse to flattery.
- Hug me, show physical affection. It opens me up to my feelings.
- I like a good discussion but not a confrontation.
- Let me know you like what I've done or said.
- Laugh with me and share in my enjoyment of life.

Relationships

Nines at their best in a relationship are kind, gentle, reassuring, supportive, loyal, and nonjudgmental.

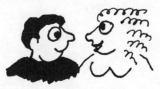

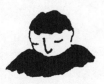

Nines at their worst in a relationship are stubborn, passive-aggressive, unassertive, overly accommodating, and defensive.

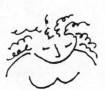

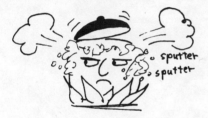

What I Like About Being a Nine

- being nonjudgmental and accepting
- caring for and being concerned about others
- being able to relax and have a good time
- knowing that most people enjoy my company; I'm easy to be around
- my ability to see many different sides of an issue and to be a good mediator and facilitator
- my heightened awareness of sensations, aesthetics, and the here and now
- being able to go with the flow and feel one with the universe

What's Hard About Being a Nine

- being judged and misunderstood for being placid and/or indecisive
- being critical of myself for lacking initiative and discipline
- being too sensitive to criticism; taking every raised eyebrow and twitch of the mouth personally
- being confused about what I really want
- caring too much about what others will think of me
- not being listened to or taken seriously

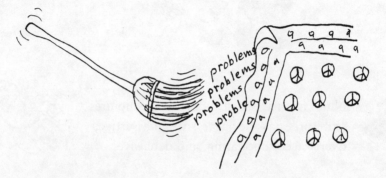

Typical Thoughts of a Nine

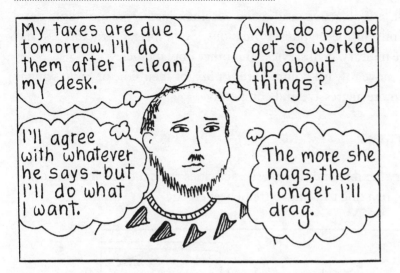

Nines as Children Often

- feel ignored and that their wants, opinions, and feelings are unimportant
- tune out a lot, especially when others argue
- are "good" children: deny anger or keep it to themselves

Nines as Parents

- are supportive, kind, and warm
- are sometimes overly permissive or nondirective

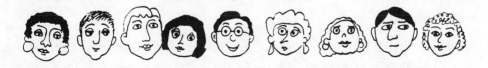

Careers

Nines listen well, are objective, and make excellent mediators and diplomats. They are frequently in the helping professions. Some prefer structured situations, such as the military, civil service, and other bureaucracies.

When Nines move toward points Three or Six, or their One or Eight wing is strong, they are more aggressive and competitive.

And Free Time

Nines can be very flexible and can pursue activities typical of each of the other eight types, from relaxing to being extremely energetic.

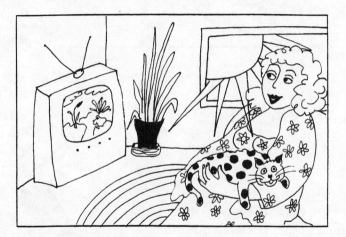

Comments About Nines

"I always feel at home and comfortable when I'm with her. She's the friend who accepts me for exactly who I am."

"My boss is the most patient and perceptive person I know. I never feel that he is judging me, which makes me want to put out all the more work."

"My friend listens to me carefully and perceives the real issues, the ones that I myself often don't see."

"My closest friend keeps me on my toes by taking me on bike trips, river rafting, whale watching, and dolphin riding. In the winter we attend lectures on the environment, peace, new scientific developments, and anthropology."

Wings

Your personality may blend into or be influenced by the types on either side of yours. A strong wing can make a big difference in your personality.

Nines with a more developed Eight wing tend to be more outgoing, assertive, and antiauthoritarian. They may vacillate between being confrontational and conciliatory.

Nines with a more developed One wing tend to be more orderly, critical, emotionally controlled, and compliant.

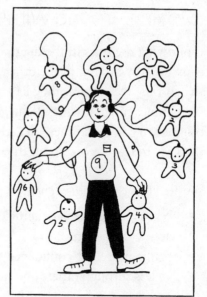

He is plugged in to everybody!

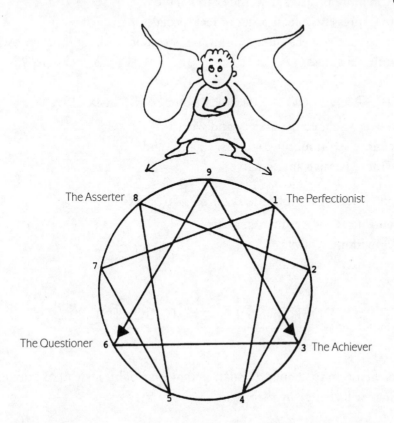

Moving Around Within the Enneagram

Following the lines in the diagram, the Nine moves toward Three in one direction and toward Six in the other. Nines move toward the positive side of Three when they feel secure; they can also consciously cultivate these positive qualities. Nines move toward the negative side of Six when in stress; they can consciously try to avoid these negative traits. Read the chapters about types Three and Six to learn more about them.

When Nines Move Toward the Positive Side of Three They
- become more energetic, efficient, and productive
- narrow their focus
- acquire more self-confidence
- live less through others and take more control of their lives

When Nines Move Toward the Negative Side of Three They
- take on more projects than they can handle
- try to impress people in order to feel special
- work to earn respect and admiration instead of working for their own meaningful goals

When Nines Move Toward the Negative Side of Six They
- become overwhelmed by anxiety and worry
- become more self-doubting, indecisive, and rigid
- become more passive and inactive

When Nines Move Toward the Positive Side of Six They
- become more direct and outspoken
- develop more loyalty
- become more practical and realistic

Practical Suggestions and Exercises for a Nine

1. Relationships
- Take the first step to change a situation that isn't right, instead of hoping that things will change by themselves.

- Ask others to join you in your interests rather than always going along with theirs.
- Bring up your problems when talking with others rather than only listening to theirs.
- Instead of answering, "I don't know" or "Whatever you want is fine with me," say, for example, "I'll let you know when I decide."
- Tell people when you want to be alone.
- Express your opinions and your feelings. Learn to rock the boat a little.

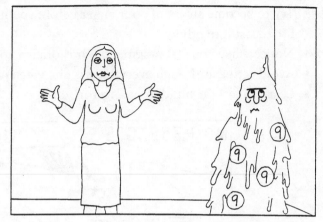

He gets into a bad mood for no apparent reason, and I'm stuck wondering why he has turned into ice!

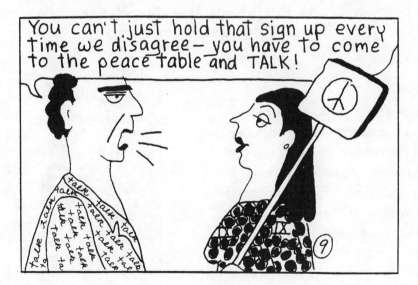

You can't just hold that sign up every time we disagree — you have to come to the peace table and TALK!

2. Anger

- Learn to become aware of, and then appropriately express, your anger. (Many Nines have volcanic outbursts as a result of repressing their anger.)

- Try to become aware of your anger before you have unknowingly broadcast it to others.
- Notice when you feel judgmental. It is often a cover-up for anger.
- Avoid acting as though everything is fine when it isn't.
- Learn to feel the buildup of anger in your body.

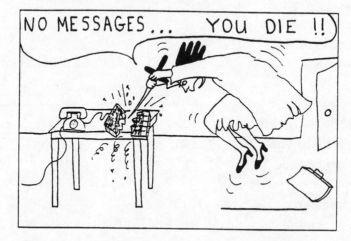

Sally is beginning to get in touch with her angry feelings.

3. Work

- Since setting goals can become a procrastination in itself, make a short list each day of what you want to accomplish. Stick to first things first.
- Set goals with definite deadlines. Set more after you have met the first.
- Take action now and deal with ambivalence and consequences later on.
- Reward yourself when you complete a task.
- Learn time-management techniques to help stay focused and on track.

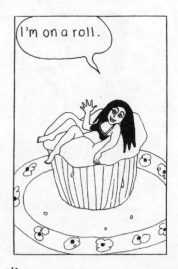

Nines can't stop once they get going.

- Lure yourself to jobs around the house by planning to listen to your favorite music while you work.

4. Procrastination and Decision Making

- Clarify your goals, since Nines can be very efficient when sure about what they want.
- If what you are contemplating feels right in your gut, do it.
- Eliminate all the things you don't want in order to help you discover what you do want.
- Make decisions based on what is pleasing to your senses: Do you like the color? How does it feel to the touch?
- Practice making decisions about small matters. Work your way up to the bigger items.

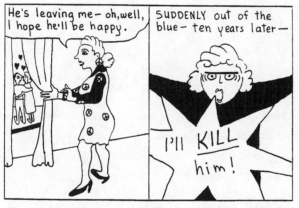

Sometimes Nines even procrastinate about blowing their tops!

5. Self-Esteem

- Engage in a physical exercise program. Tai chi and other martial arts are especially good for Nines.
- Resist distracting yourself from your problems with food, drugs, television, oversleeping, or reading.
- When a relationship ends, resist the temptation to start another one right away. Spend some time reflecting on the strengths and weaknesses of the relationship.

- In order to develop independence, establish other friendships and connections in addition to your partner.
- When you have problems, ask a friend just to listen and give you no advice.

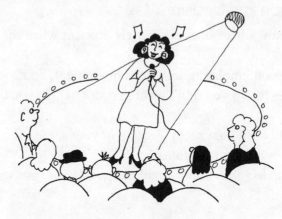

Display your talents—let us enjoy your gifts.

Things Nines Would Never Dream of Doing

- complying immediately when their partner tells them to do an unpleasant job in an authoritarian manner
- calling up an aggressive talk-show host and engaging in a screaming match
- purposefully creating an uproar at a family gathering

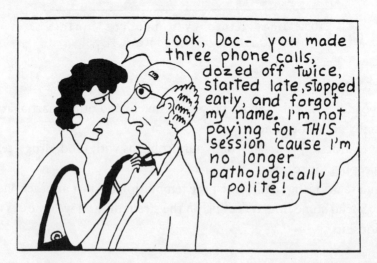

Look, Doc— you made three phone calls, dozed off twice, started late, stopped early, and forgot my name. I'm not paying for THIS session 'cause I'm no longer pathologically polite!

- announcing long ahead of time that they are going somewhere they know their partner won't approve of, so the partner will have plenty of time to fight with them about it
- telling everyone in a group they are angry and exactly what each person there did to make them so
- saying, "I don't want to talk," when a friend who desperately needs sympathy calls up
- confronting someone face-to-face in an extremely critical manner

Positive Things to Say to Yourself

I will ask for what I want.

I will learn to recognize my resentment and use it as a source of energy.

I will even let myself feel guilty rather than rush to fulfill another's expectations.

I have what it takes. I am enough.

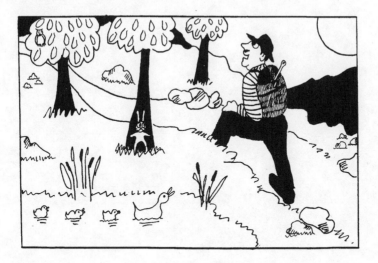

AFTER THE DINNER PARTY

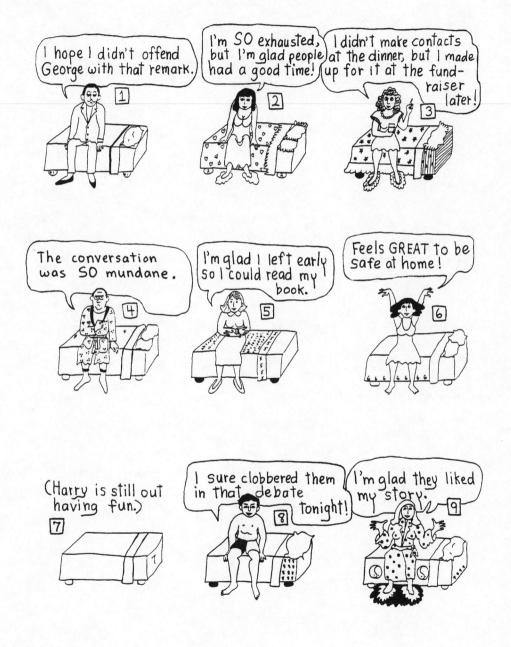

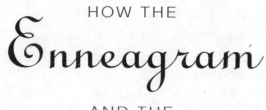

HOW THE
Enneagram
AND THE
Jungian Types
Fit Together

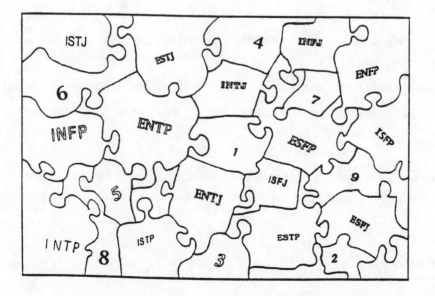

Many of the variations within the nine types can be explained by relating the highly respected Myers-Briggs Type Indicator (the MBTI) to the Enneagram. This will increase accuracy, give greater breadth to the system, and lead to a more finely tuned understanding of ourselves and others. You do not need to already know the MBTI system, since we will familiarize you with it here. We will

- define the eight MBTI preferences
- apply these eight preferences to the Enneagram types
- explain each of the sixteen MBTI personalities within the context of Keirsey's four temperaments
- correlate the two systems in a useful chart

Introduction to the MBTI* Personality Inventory

It is believed that we are born with a preference for four of the eight personality traits that the MBTI measures (one from each of four pairs). In the first half of life, we strengthen these preferred traits in order to build a strong personality. In the second half of life, we strengthen the weaker traits and become more balanced and whole. For example, an introvert may develop more extroversion and an extrovert may develop more introversion.

The Myers Briggs Type Indicator is a personality inventory or test based on the work of Carl G. Jung. It measures individual preferences on these four scales:

1. whether people relate more to the external or internal world (*Extroversion* or *Introversion*)

2. how people prefer to take in or perceive information (*Sensing* or *iNtuition*)

3. how people prefer to make evaluations and decisions (*Thinking* or *Feeling*)

   and

4. how people live: whether they are organized and seek closure or are spontaneous and open (*Judging* or *Perceiving*)

---

*Isabel Myers and her mother, Katharine Briggs, created the MBTI and added the Perceiving and Judging preferences to Jung's types.

Each four-letter type consists of a combination of one preference from each of the above pairs of traits. A person who prefers *Extroversion*, *Sensing*, *Thinking*, and *Judging* is referred to as an *ESTJ*. There are sixteen possible combinations or types.

Although we use all eight preferences, one in each pair tends to be more developed.

MBTI Definitions

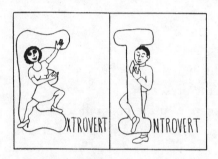

The Extroverted and Introverted Preferences
Whether people relate more to the external or internal world.

Extroverts

- are outgoing, active, and tend to feel at ease with people
- get energized by the outer world
- are interested in the breadth of experiences
- discover what they think and feel by talking and doing
- act first and perhaps reflect on it later

Introverts

- are quiet and reflective and prefer relating one to one
- get energized by being alone
- are interested in the depth of experience
- discover what they think and feel by processing information internally
- reflect first, then perhaps act

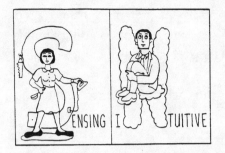

The Sensing and iNtuitive Preferences

How people take in or perceive information.

Sensates

- rely on information obtained directly through their five senses
- are practical and down to earth; live in the present
- are interested in what is at hand more than in future possibilities
- work step-by-step in an established way; usually pay attention to details

iNtuitives (abbreviated by *N*)

- obtain information through their sixth sense of hunches, insights, and inspirations
- are interested in possibilities; use their imagination and vision
- like doing things in new ways; work in bursts of energy
- focus on the big picture; tend to ignore details

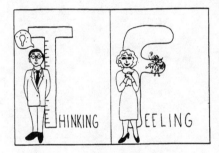

The Thinking and Feeling Preferences

Once people have perceived information through their Sensing and iNtuitive preferences, they come to conclusions and make decisions based on their Thinking and Feeling preferences.

Thinkers

- use logic and analysis to make decisions
- value principles, laws, and procedures
- tend to be impersonal, objective, and critical

Feelers

- filter information through their personal values
- value harmony; are supportive and empathic
- thrive on praise; are sensitive to criticism

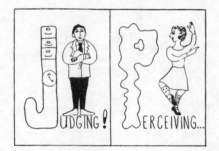

The Judging and Perceiving Preferences

This measures how people organize their lives when relating to the outside world. Judgers make relatively quick value judgments using Thinking or Feeling in order to come to closure. Perceivers put off closure while collecting information through their Sensing and iNtuition.

Judgers

- are relatively structured and efficient
- live in a planned and organized way; tend to make lists and follow them
- push for decisions quickly in order to have closure

Having a preference for Judging does not mean being "judgmental."

Perceivers

- are relatively adaptable, flexible, and spontaneous
- want to keep their options open and explore new possibilities
- postpone closure by taking in more and more information before making decisions

The Jungian Preferences
Applied to the Enneagram

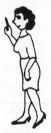

One
(The Perfectionist)

Extroverted Ones are often leaders and tend to impose their standards of perfection on others.

Introverted Ones direct their perfectionism inward and tend to focus on improving themselves.

Sensate Ones are practical and detail oriented and value rules and traditions.

iNtuitive Ones tend to be idealistic, innovative, individualistic, and nontraditional.

Thinking Ones are logical, analytical, critical, and more concerned with data and things than with people.

Feeling Ones value helping people, foster harmony, are more fearful of criticism, and are more likely to turn their anger inward.

Their usual preference for *Judging* means that *Ones* are dependable, organized, and structured.

Developing *Perceiving* makes *Ones* more flexible, adaptable, and spontaneous.

The predominant feature of Ones is Judging.

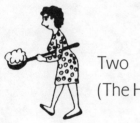

Two
(The Helper)

Extroverted Twos are talkative, dramatic, and energetic. They reach out to people and like receiving attention.

Introverted Twos are more reserved and quietly helpful.

Sensate Twos offer practical, down-to-earth help to others.

iNtuitive Twos are more individualistic and live more in the world of ideas. They develop the art of persuasion and think of possibilities that would improve people's lives.

Twos prefer *Feeling*. They are usually warm and empathic and strive to make their environment harmonious.

Developing the *Thinking* qualities of objectivity and detachment helps the *Two* take things less personally. Twos are almost never Thinking types.

Judging Twos are conscientious, serious, orderly, and responsible.

Perceiving Twos tend to be more lighthearted, adaptable, and spontaneous.

The predominant feature of Twos is Feeling. They tend toward Extroversion.

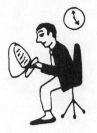

Three
(The Achiever)

Threes tend to be *Extroverted,* action oriented, and fast paced. Extroverted Threes are good communicators and like to be in the limelight.

Introverted Threes are quieter, more reserved, and inner-focused.

Sensate Threes tend to be realistic, traditional, detail-oriented problem solvers.

Intuitive Threes are future oriented and innovative or visionary.

Threes who prefer *Thinking* are objective, tough-minded, and goal oriented. They are likely to become heads of organizations.

Feeling Threes are more people oriented and more likely to be women. Harmony is very important to them.

Judging Threes are structured, organized, and efficient.

Perceiving Threes are more spontaneous, flexible, and adaptable.

Threes tend toward Extroversion and Judging.

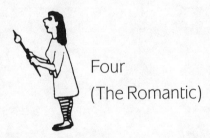

Four
(The Romantic)

Extroverted Fours are sociable and expressive (sometimes flamboyant). They are likely to have a more developed Three wing.

Introverted Fours are more serious, reserved, and withdrawn.

Sensate Fours express themselves through action and live more in the here and now.

iNtuitive Fours are insightful, idealistic, and often more interested in the world of imagination than in everyday reality.

Fours prefer *Feeling*. They are emotionally sensitive, empathic, and warm.

Thinking Fours are rare. They tend to be more analytical and objective.

Judging helps *Fours* to focus and persevere.

Perceiving Fours are more impulsive, indecisive, and adaptable.

The predominant features of Fours are Introversion and Feeling.

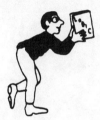

Five
(The Observer)

Extroverted Fives are outspoken, sociable, and intellectually assertive.

Most *Fives* are *Introverted* and detached, reserved, and quiet.

Sensate Fives are realistic, practical, and like to classify data.

iNtuitive Fives tend to be more insightful, innovative, theoretical, and scholarly.

Thinking Fives use logic and analysis to solve problems and make decisions.

Feeling Fives tend to be sensitive and tuned in to people; they probably have a more developed Four wing.

Judging Fives are organized, determined, and tend to put their ideas out into the world.

Perceiving Fives are less focused on completion. They can get sidetracked by other possibilities.

The predominant features of Fives are Introversion and Thinking.

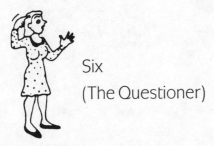

Six
(The Questioner)

(Sixes tend to swing back and forth between preferences more than any other type.)

Extroverted Sixes are talkative and sociable.

Introverted Sixes are more reserved and private.

Sensate Sixes are practical, dependable, and traditional.

Intuitive Sixes are more individualistic, innovative, and future oriented. They prefer talking and thinking to action.

Thinking Sixes tend to be critical, objective, and logical. They are more likely to be counterphobic than the Feeling types.

Feeling Sixes are caring, loyal, dependent, and tend to be phobic.

Sixes often prefer *Judging*. They value structure and closure.

Perceiving Sixes are more adaptable and spontaneous.

Sixes correlate with every MBTI type.

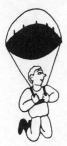

Seven
(The Adventurer)

Extroverted Sevens are talkative, sociable, fast paced, and fun loving. They usually have a large variety of friends and experiences.

Introverted Sevens are more reserved, private, and quietly playful.

Sensate Sevens are action oriented, playful, and realistic. They learn from first-hand experience and observation.

Intuitive Sevens tend to be imaginative, creative, and innovative.

Thinking Sevens tend to be objective, logical, challenging, and blunt.

Feeling Sevens are gentler, more sympathetic, and more people oriented.

Judging Sevens tend to be good administrators and organizers with excellent follow-through on projects and plans.

Sevens often prefer *Perceiving*. They like to keep their options open and sometimes have difficulty seeing projects through to the end.

Sevens tend toward Extroversion and Perceiving.

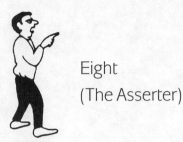

Eight
(The Asserter)

Extroverted Eights are energetic, exuberant, outspoken, and fast paced. They often become forceful leaders.

Introverted Eights are private, reserved, and quietly controlling. They appear quite different from Extroverted Eights.

Sensate Eights tend to be down to earth, pragmatic, and interested in facts.

Intuitive Eights tend to become visionary or innovative leaders.

Eights who prefer *Thinking* are direct, analytical, and blunt.

Eights who prefer *Feeling* are helpful and supportive. They are less forceful or controlling than Thinking Eights unless pushed or treated unfairly.

Eights who prefer *Judging* are decisive, organized, and persevering.

Eights who prefer *Perceiving* are more spontaneous, restless, and antiauthoritarian.

Eights tend toward Extroversion and Thinking.

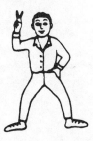

Nine
(The Peacemaker)

Extroverted Nines are sociable, talkative, and energetic.

Introverted Nines are quietly friendly, modest, and reserved.

Sensate Nines are traditional, down to earth, and live in the moment.

iNtuitive Nines are more idealistic, individualistic, and interested in the world of ideas and possibilities.

Nines who prefer *Thinking* tend to be analytical, critical, and objective.

Nines who prefer *Feeling* value harmony and pleasant relationships.

Judging Nines are organized and productive and want closure.

Nines are often *Perceivers*. They like to keep their options open and can have difficulty with completion.

Nines tend toward Introversion and Perceiving.

The Enneagram Correlated with the Sixteen Myers-Briggs Types

(Organized According to David Keirsey's Theory of "Four Temperaments")

Traditionalists: The SJ Temperament

Sensate Judgers

- want to be useful, to serve others, and to belong
- are dutiful, loyal, and conscientious; they value family and tradition
- are realistic and practical; they like structure and clearly defined procedures
- often worry about the future
- can feel obligated, overburdened, and taken for granted

Careers: working for established institutions and serving others as teachers, managers, nurses, preachers, bankers, salespeople, civil service workers, and homemakers.

ESTJs (Extroversion Sensing Thinking Judging) are logical, decisive, efficient, and outspoken; they want to be in charge and they value efficiency.

ESFJs (Extroversion Sensing Feeling Judging) are enthusiastic, warm, talkative, and sympathetic; they want to be of service to others.

ISTJs (Introversion Sensing Thinking Judging) are quiet, serious, exacting, and hardworking; they are detail oriented and strong in follow-through.

ISFJs (Introversion Sensing Feeling Judging) are quietly friendly, modest, devoted, and unusually dependable. They often help others behind the scenes.

Action Oriented: The SP Temperament

Sensate Perceivers

- like freedom and action yet are practical and realistic
- are optimistic, generous, enthusiastic, spontaneous, and flexible
- are "free spirits" and want to be seen as such; they don't like confinement, obligation, or routine
- live in and enjoy the present; they are not as interested in long-range plans and completion

Careers: like variety and challenge as pilots, firefighters, paramedics, entrepreneurs, troubleshooters, and athletes. Some like working as contractors, craftspeople, performers, nurses, teachers, and child-care workers.

ESTPs (Extroversion Sensing Thinking Perceiving) are pragmatic, energetic, attracted to risk and challenge, and are sometimes blunt and outrageous.

ESFPs (Extroversion Sensing Feeling Perceiving) are friendly, easygoing, gregarious, and talkative; they enjoy helping others.

ISTPs (Introversion Sensing Thinking Perceiving) are quiet, reserved, independent, detached, and often curious onlookers.

ISFPs (Introversion Sensing Feeling Perceiving) are natural, gentle, modest, loyal, compassionate, open-minded, and conciliatory.

Knowledge Seekers: The NT Temperament

iNtuitive Thinkers

- have the need to know and to be competent
- are innovative, analytical, and theoretical
- are interested in the big picture, in what could or might be
- place high demands on themselves
- often challenge authorities or test the system

Careers: exploring ideas, developing models, building systems as scientists, philosophers, architects, inventors, engineers, security analysts.

ENTJs (Extroversion iNtuition Thinking Judging) are innovative, logical, efficient, direct, decisive, and demanding; they often become leaders.

ENTPs (Extroversion iNtuition Thinking Perceiving) are enthusiastic, outspoken, nonconforming, innovative, and ingenious; they can have difficulty with follow-through.

INTJs (Introversion iNtuition Thinking Judging) are very independent, determined, and individualistic. They drive themselves and others to meet goals.

INTPs (Introversion iNtuition Thinking Perceiving) are theoretical, analytical, curious, reserved, and insightful. They value precision in thought and language and like to solve problems.

Identity Seekers: The NF Temperament

iNtuitive Feelers

- seek and express an identity that is uniquely their own; they are imaginative and insightful and the least understood by others
- are warm and caring; they invest a lot of themselves in relationships
- are easily hurt by criticism
- value bettering the world and bringing out the best in people; they look for new possibilities to help others reach their potential

Careers: good at inspiring and persuading through speaking, writing, or creating as novelists, journalists, teachers, salespeople, artists, actors, actresses, and counselors.

ENFJs (*Extroversion iNtuition Feeling Judging*) are exuberant, curious, friendly, sympathetic, helpful, and conscientious; they make gifted speakers and leaders.

ENFPs (*Extroversion iNtuition Feeling Perceiving*) are enthusiastic, imaginative, versatile, and good at communicating and thinking up possibilities. They start projects enthusiastically but tend to move on before completing them.

INFJs (*Introversion iNtuition Feeling Judging*) are gentle, quiet, conscientious, persevering, and seek harmony with others. They are quietly forceful regarding their principles and ideals.

INFPs (*Introversion iNtuition Feeling Perceiving*) are reserved, gentle, curious, creative, open-minded, and idealistic. They often prefer working independently.

Enneagram Types

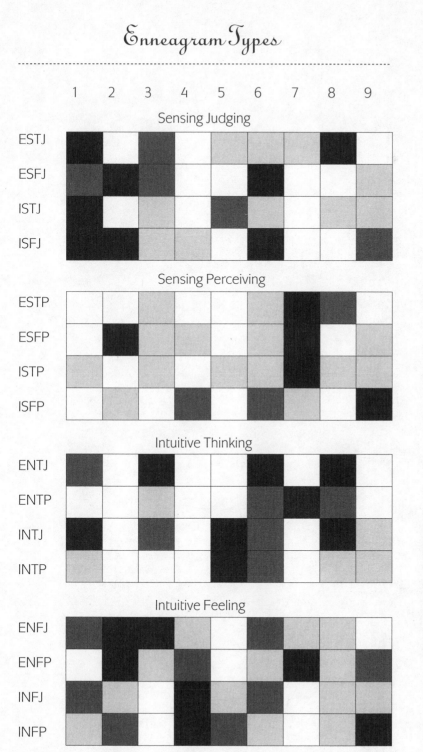

	1	2	3	4	5	6	7	8	9

Sensing Judging

ESTJ									
ESFJ									
ISTJ									
ISFJ									

Sensing Perceiving

ESTP									
ESFP									
ISTP									
ISFP									

Intuitive Thinking

ENTJ									
ENTP									
INTJ									
INTP									

Intuitive Feeling

ENFJ									
ENFP									
INFJ									
INFP									

Most Common

Quite Common

Less Common

Least Common

Suggested Reading

Enneagram Books

Hurley, Kathleen V., and Theodore E. Dobson. *What's My Type?* San Francisco: HarperSanFrancisco, 1992.

Palmer, Helen. *The Enneagram*. San Francisco: HarperSanFrancisco, 1991.

Riso, Don Richard. *Personality Types*. Boston: Houghton Mifflin Co., 1987.

———. *Understanding the Enneagram*. Boston: Houghton Mifflin Co., 1990.

———. *Discovering Your Personality Type*. Boston: Houghton Mifflin Co., 1992.

———. *Enneagram Transformations*. Boston: Houghton Mifflin Co., 1993.

Rohr, Richard, and Andreas Ebert. *Discovering The Enneagram*. Crossroad Publishing Company, 1990.

Myers-Briggs Books

Hirsh, Sandra, and Jean Kummerow. *Life Types*. New York: Warner Books, 1989.

Keirsey, David, and Marilyn Bates. *Please Understand Me*. Del Mar, CA: Prometheus Nemesis Book Co., 1978.

Kroeger, Otto, and Janet Thuesen. *Type Talk*. New York: Delacorte, 1988.

Myers, Isabel Briggs, and Peter B. Myers. *Gifts Differing*. Palo Alto, CA: Consulting Psychologists Press, 1980.

For Other Enneagram Resources (Tapes, Books, Publications)

Credence Cassettes, 115 E. Armour Blvd., P.O. Box 419491, Kansas City, MO, 64141–6491

The Changeworks Catalogue, P.O. Box 1066, Portland, OR, 97210–0612

Acknowledgments

Thanks to:

John Loudon—our editor at Harper

Dorothy Wall—for her advice and encouragement

Linda Allen—our agent

Our Enneagram teachers:

Helen Palmer for her book and her panels, which made the types come to life
Don Riso for his rich, clear books
Our other teachers: Richard Rohr, Thomas Condon, Rich Byrne, and Michael Gardner
And our Myers-Briggs teachers, including David Keirsey and Joyce Beckett

Those we interviewed for this book:

Eve Abbott	Peter Blakey	Susan Brown
John Argue	Sam Blood	David Burke
Timothy Baron-O'Hagain	Ed Bourne	Judy Burke
Laurie Bates	Julie Brook	Joyce Burks
Sondra Beck	Bob Brown	Claudia Cadwell
Joseph Benenfeld	Christopher Brown	Jerry Cavanaugh
Shirley Benenfeld	Corky Brown	Ragan Cavanaugh
Sarah Berger	Lois Brown	Sandra Cobb
Eloise Bergesen	Nancy Brown	John Costarella

Karen Costarella
Patricia Craven
Mary Beth Crenna
Madonna Datzman
Devah De Fusco
Helen Del Tredici
Penny De Wind
Tom Draper
Dan Dunn
Christian Eddelman
Victoria Eddelman
Ben Eiland
Annette Evenary
Gloria Everett
Sylvia Falcon
Christine Federici
Mani Feniger
Mara Fine
Shiela Fish
Dan Fivey
Teri Fivey
Susan Flatmo
Francine Foltz
Gary Foltz
Janet Forman
Ken Forman
Peg Freda
Lee Anna Friedman
Renee Gamez
Harry Gans
Dori Geller
Phil Gerrard
Harriet Berman Glaser
Lee Glickstein
Al Gould
Kathleen Greaves
Janice Heidmiller
Eleanor Henderson
Richard Hendrickson

Joan Hitlin
Holly Holmes
Katya Hope
Marybeth Hudson
Bonnie Isaacs
Fred Isaacs
Juliette Jacque
Margery Jamison
Surja Jessup
Susan Johnson
Chinabear Joseph
Mark Kanat
Nancy Kanat
Tish Kanat
Donna Kaufman
Nancy Kesselring
Premseri Khalsa
Shakti Singh Khalsa
Stephen Kresge
Lolli Levine
Ginny Logan
David Luke
Vivienne Luke
Ellen Lynch
Karen Tussing McArdle
Alison McCabe
Marilyn McNamara
Janet Manfield
Howard Margolis
Carolina Marks
Steven Marks
Rebecca Mayeno
Helen Meyer
John Meyer
Joan Mitlin
Con Mondfrans
Ed Mooney
Marla Morton
Debby Nakamura

Dennis Nakamura
Trevor Nelson
Ellen Odza
Fran Packard
Sita Packer
Patricia Padgett
Susan Page
Felice Pearl
Suzanne Pereira
Linda Petty
Barbara Pichotto
Pamela Pitts
Jim Popf
Scott Ramsey
Janice Fuller Ravitz
Bertha Reilly
Madeleine Reilly
Winifred Reilly
Guinn Rigsby
Shankiri Rise
Tricia Rissman
Peter Rogers
Helga Romoser
Loie Rosenkrantz
Tom Rosin
Gail Royce
Helen Rubardt
Ken Rubardt
Tom Rucker
Lucienne Sanchez-Resnik
Beth Sanguinetti
David Sapper
Juditte Schwartz
Maylie Scott
Jo Sherrill
Rosie Sorenson
Robert Sprague
John Stedman
Ellen Strong

Annemarie Sudermann
Greg Supriano
Bill Swahlen
Duncan Tam
Toni Tischler
Linda Tobin
Elisa Trevisani
Ann Underhill Tussing
Catherine Minor Valdez

Robert Valdez
Noni Verbiscar-Brown
Ram Vignola
August F. Wagele
Dorothy Wagele
Jim Wagele
Joan Wagele
Susan Weinstein
Elin Weiss

Eileen Williams
Judy Wolberg
Ann Woodward
George Woodward
Steve Woolpert
Gail Wread
Marcie Zellner
Victoria Zenoff

About the Authors

Renee Baron is a writer and uses the
Enneagram in her counseling practice.

Elizabeth Wagele is a writer
and professional cartoonist.

Both live in Berkeley, CA.

Other Books on the Enneagram
available from Harper San Francisco:
....

The Enneagram: Understanding Yourself and the Others in Your Life by Helen Palmer
*The Enneagram in Love & Work: Understanding Your Intimate & Business
    Relationships* by Helen Palmer
*What's My Type?: Using the Enneagram System of Nine Personality Types to Discover
    Your Best Self* by Kathleen V. Hurley and Theodore E. Dobson
My Best Self: Using the Enneagram to Free the Soul by Kathleen V. Hurley and
    Theodore E. Dobson

(1) Perfectionist - 4
(2) Helper - 7
(3) Achiever - 1
(4) Romantic - 10 *
(5) Observer - 13 *
(6) Questioner - 3
(7) Adventurer - 8
(8) Asserter - 6
(9) Peacemaker - 11 *